Racial, ethnic, and socioeconomic disparities exist in the prevalence and treatment of OM in children. Smith and Boss performed a systematic review concluding that disparities exist for the prevalence and treatment of OM in children in the United States, especially for surgical treatment.[18]

Pacifier use has been theorized to increase the risk of AOM. Niemela and colleagues hypothesized that pacifier use increased the annual incidence of AOM and calculated that pacifier use was responsible for 25% of AOM episodes in children younger than 3 years. They performed an intervention trial by randomizing various well-child clinics to either receive education that pacifier use should be limited or where this information was not provided. The group provided with the pacifier information had a 29% decrease in AOM. The mechanistic theories are that the sucking action of the child propels nasopharyngeal secretions into the middle ear or that the pacifier acts as a fomite. The exact role and contribution of pacifier use in AOM remains unclear.[5,19]

PATHOPHYSIOLOGY AND PATHOGENESIS
Eustachian Tube Dysfunction

The Eustachian tube in the infant is less effective at ventilating the middle ear and is structurally shorter, wider, and more horizontal than in the adult; this leads to the higher prevalence of OM in infants and young children. The Eustachian tube has a more adult configuration by age 7 years, and the prevalence of OM is much lower by this age.[5,20] Typically as a child ages, OME is more likely to resolve spontaneously. One study found that spontaneous resolution of OME occurred in 22% of cases at 1 year, 37% at 2 years, 50% at 3 years, 60% at 4 years, 70% at 5 years, 85% at 7 years, and 95% at 10 years.[21,22]

Bluestone and Klein described 3 physiologic functions of the Eustachian tube: (1) pressure regulation or ventilation, (2) protection, and (3) clearance or drainage. Of these 3 functions, pressure regulation is deemed the most important. Middle ear pressure equilibrates to atmospheric pressure through a series of active intermittent openings of the Eustachian tube. Contractions of the tensor veli palatini muscle during swallowing, jaw movements, or yawning transiently open the tube. If there is any impairment of Eustachian tube function, the likelihood of negative pressure developing in the middle ear is high. Regulation of pressure can be impaired by either functional or anatomic obstruction. In ears with normal Eustachian tube function, the tube is collapsed at rest, protecting the middle ear from the reflux of nasopharyngeal secretions. The clearance of secretions produced in the middle ear into the nasopharynx is accomplished via the mucociliary system and through the "pumping action" of the Eustachian tube. The passive closing of the tube is initiated at the middle ear end of the Eustachian tube and progresses toward the nasopharynx, which results in removal of the secretion.[5,10]

Infection

Before the introduction of the vaccines against *Streptococcus pneumoniae*, it was the most common bacterial pathogen in AOM, followed by *Haemophilus influenzae* and *Moraxella catarrhalis*. Over time, there was a documented shift to serotypes of *S pneumoniae* that were not covered in any vaccine and then, ultimately, a decrease in *S pneumoniae* AOM infections compared with other bacterial pathogens. *H influenzae* is now the most frequent bacterial isolate from MEE. The presence of biofilms may also contribute to resistant episodes of AOM. Biofilms are sessile communities of interacting bacteria attached to a surface and encased in a matrix that bestows protection from phagocytosis and other host defense mechanisms. The reduced metabolic rate of bacteria in the biofilm renders them resistant to antimicrobial treatment. Post and colleagues, using PCR methodology, found evidence of bacteria in 48% of culture-negative MEEs from children undergoing TTP for chronic OME.[23] Certain viruses have been isolated from MEE, specifically respiratory syncytial virus (RSV), influenza, adenovirus, parainfluenza, and rhinovirus.[15,24] There is strong evidence that viruses play an important role in the pathogenesis of AOM. In most children, a viral URI initiates the cascade of events that ultimately causes an AOM.

Even though allergy is considered in the pathogenesis of OM, the relationship is unclear. Treatment with allergy medications has not shown efficacy as OM therapy. Proposed mechanisms whereby allergy may contribute to OM include (1) the middle ear as a shock organ (target), (2) allergy-induced inflammatory swelling of the Eustachian tube mucosa, (3) inflammatory obstruction of the nose, and (4) aspiration of bacteria-laden allergic nasopharyngeal secretions into the middle ear. Most of the proposed mechanisms report a relationship between allergy and abnormal Eustachian tube function. Prospective studies confirm this relationship by performing a series of provocative, intranasal, allergen-inhalation challenge studies.[25] Children with major immune deficiencies may have RAOM as part of their overall clinical picture, but children who are otitis-prone may only have a subtle immunologic abnormality that predisposes them to recurrent infections.[26] Children with Eustachian tube dysfunction and low immunoglobulin A (IgA) or low IgG2 and decreased levels of mannose-binding lecithin have been shown to have high rates of recurrence of bilateral OME after TTP.[27]

Gastroesophageal reflux (GER) or laryngopharyngeal reflux (LPR) has been hypothesized to contribute to the incidence of OM in children. Two recent studies, a systematic review by Lechien and colleagues and a meta-analysis by Wu and colleagues had contrasting conclusions as to the association of reflux and OM. Lechien and colleagues found that the prevalence of LPR and GER in patients with OM were 28.7% and 40.7%, respectively. Most of the studies identified pepsin or pepsinogen in MEE but with a range of mean concentrations depending on the pH measurement technique. The definitions of COME, RAOM, and LPR was heterogenous depending on the study. They concluded that the association between LPR and OM remains unclear.[28] Wu and colleagues identified a significant relationship between OME and GER with a pooled odds ratio of 4.52. Their meta-analysis suggested a significant association between OME and GER.[29] Such disparate conclusions based on potentially overlapping data warrant additional research.

Prevention of Disease

Management of environmental factors
The incidence of OM may be decreased if breastfeeding in the first 6 months of life is promoted and supine bottle feeding and pacifier use are avoided. Elimination of passive tobacco smoke and alteration of child care arrangements would also decrease the risk of developing AOM.[5]

Vaccines
The 3 most common bacteria isolated from MEE are S pneumoniae, H influenzae, and M catarrhalis. Pneumovax, Prevnar, and Prevnar 13 are vaccines against S pneumoniae and have shown great success at decreasing the frequency of AOM episodes caused by this bacterium. Studies showed that immunized children were 20% less likely to require TTP. Additional follow-up of study subjects continued to demonstrate a modest amount of protection against episodes of AOM and TTP.[30]

Viral vaccines have the potential to act at an earlier stage in the pathogenesis of OM. They may prevent viral URIs and ultimately prevent AOM episodes. Norhayati and colleagues performed a systematic review to assess the effectiveness of the influenza vaccine in reducing the occurrence of AOM in infants and children, concluding that the influenza vaccine results in a small reduction in AOM. The corresponding reduction in antibiotic usage needs to be considered in light of current recommendations aimed at avoiding antibiotic overuse.[31] Especially for younger children, Synagis, which is a vaccine against RSV, can be helpful at preventing both lower airway infections and episodes of AOM.

TREATMENT
Acute Otitis Media

In the report from the American Academy of Pediatrics Subcommittee on Management of Acute Otitis Media, published in 2004, an observation strategy was recommended as a viable option in the management of AOM, depending on the age of the patient, severity of the disease, diagnostic certainty, and access to medical care.[32] Severe disease is defined as moderate-to-severe otalgia, fever greater than 39° C (102° F) orally, or a toxic appearing child. Children younger than 6 months should always be treated with antibiotics. Healthy children between 6 and 23 months of age with nonsevere disease and an uncertain diagnosis could be observed, but if the AOM is certain or severe, the child should be treated with antibiotics. Children older than 23 months could be observed if the AOM is not severe or the diagnosis is uncertain but treated if the AOM is severe. If the appropriate close clinical follow-up is in question or if access to medical care is limited, the AOM should be treated (**Fig. 2**). The Management Guidelines strongly recommended adequate treatment to reduce pain in children with an AOM. The appropriate choice of oral antibiotics for AOM depends greatly on the diagnostic accuracy and the ability to distinguish AOM from OME. For nonsevere episodes of AOM, amoxicillin, 90 mg/kg/d, in 2 divided doses is the first-line therapy, primarily to cover *S pneumonia*. For severe episodes of AOM, amoxicillin/clavulanate (amoxicillin, 90 mg/kg/d, and clavulanic acid, 6.4 mg/kg/d, in 2 divided doses) is recommended and should provide adequate coverage for beta-

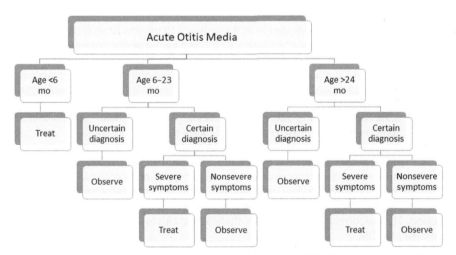

Fig. 2. Algorithm for the treatment of acute otitis media (AOM). Treatment for an AOM is determined by the age of the patient, the certainty of diagnosis, and the severity of the symptoms. For any age, the accessibility of healthcare for follow up evaluations must be considered.

lactamase producing *H influenza* and *M catarrhalis*. Cephalosporins should only be considered as first-line treatment in children who have a penicillin allergy. Typically, a 10-day course of antibiotics is prescribed and has been shown to reduce the number of early treatment failures in younger children.[10] Decongestants, antihistamines, and steroids may provide variable short-term symptomatic relief in some patients but have not been shown to provide any improvement in clinical outcome. In fact, the high potential for adverse effects caused by these medications makes the risk outweigh the benefit in this patient population.

Complications of acute otitis media

Complications of AOM are most commonly suppurative with spread of the infection beyond the middle ear space. Mattos and colleagues reported on the intratemporal and intracranial complications of AOM, noting that the most of the complications were intratemporal, with 86.1% presenting with acute mastoiditis, 38% with subperiosteal abscess, and 16.7% with facial nerve palsy. More rare complications included sigmoid sinus thrombosis in 8.3% of patients and epidural abscess in 7.4%. Other patients had otitic hydrocephalus, internal jugular thrombosis, and Gradenigo syndrome with abducens palsy. Cultures grew *S pneumoniae* in one-third of patients and, of those, more than half were multidrug resistant. Nearly all patients with subperiosteal abscess underwent mastoid surgery as did 8 of 10 patients with epidural abscess in addition to incision and drainage of the abscess.[33]

Recurrent Acute Otitis Media

Medical treatment

The administration of prophylactic, longer term antibiotics may decrease the number of episodes of AOM in children who are prone to infections; this may be a helpful treatment course for children who are at high risk for surgical intervention or general anesthesia. Leach and Morris reviewed all randomized controlled trials of long-term antibiotics versus placebo for the prevention of AOM, AOM with perforation, or CSOM. They concluded that long-term antibiotics reduced any episode of AOM and the number of episodes of AOM. Approximately 5 children would need to be treated long term to prevent one child from experiencing an AOM during treatment. Antibiotics prevented 1.5 episodes of AOM for every 12 months of treatment per child. Antibiotic use was not associated with a significant increase in adverse events. They concluded that for children at risk, antibiotics given once or twice daily reduced the probability of AOM during treatment. Antibiotics reduce the number of episodes of AOM per year from around 3 to around 1.5. The larger benefit is bestowed on children at highest risk for RAOM.[34]

Other complementary and alternative medicine (CAM) treatment options that are given or performed in an effort to prevent AOM were studied by Marom and colleagues but found that supporting evidence was lacking and recommended against considering them as potential treatment of AOM. They performed a systematic review of CAM treatments, such as acupuncture, homeopathy, herbal medicine/phytotherapy, osteopathy, chiropractic, xylitol, ear candling, vitamin D supplements, and systemic and topical probiotics. They reviewed each treatment and found supportive evidence lacking. They recommended additional studies to evaluate the potential value of CAM therapies for OM.[35]

Surgical treatment

In children who have persistent AOM despite maximal medical therapy, including high-dose amoxicillin/clavulanate and intramuscular ceftriaxone, may benefit from a myringotomy or tympanocentesis in the office setting. Decompression of the bulging

TM relieves the pain and, most importantly, allows for any antibiotic course to be culture driven. If such an infection has not been an isolated event, a more urgent TTP with cultures taken in the operating room can be considered. Although at potentially higher risk of postoperative otorrhea, the ability to administer ototopical medications to treat the infection is an important benefit.

Although the mainstay surgical treatment of RAOM is TTP, there are important considerations. The criteria for TTP for RAOM is for 3 or more AOM episodes in 6 months or 4 or more AOM episodes in 12 months with one infection being recent. There must also be an MEE present at the time of the clinic examination when tube placement is considered. The 2013 Clinical Practice Guideline: Tympanostomy Tubes in Children very clearly assert that clinicians should not perform TTP in children with RAOM who do not have an MEE at the time of assessment for tube candidacy. Further, the guideline states that clinicians should determine if a child with RAOM or OME of any duration is at increased risk for speech, language, or learning problems from OM because of baseline sensory, physical, cognitive, or behavioral factors.[36] TTP may be underutilized in children who are deemed "at risk" for behavioral or learning concerns because OME is often asymptomatic, and the uncooperative child can be difficult to examine to confirm the presence of MEE.[37]

Adenoidectomy in the treatment of ear disease can be a helpful adjunct to TTP. The rationale for removal of the adenoids is that large adenoids obstruct the nasopharynx and, consequently, the Eustachian tube, preventing ventilation of the middle ear and mastoid system.[38] Further, adenoid tissue in children with OM may have increased bacterial colonization,[39] which may predispose to recurrent infections. Coticchia and colleagues demonstrated that the adenoids are covered with biofilm and may act as a reservoir for bacteria, which can then cause middle ear disease.[40] The effect of adenoidectomy on OM is independent of adenoid size. Adenoidectomy may provide modest improvement in children with RAOM but is not recommended as a first-line procedure unless it is otherwise indicated for airway obstruction.

Otitis Media with Effusion

OM with effusion (OME) is defined as fluid in the middle ear space without any associated signs or symptoms of infection. OME is frequently diagnosed in early childhood with one study finding OME in 50% of children younger than 1 year and in 60% of children younger than 2 years. The first step in the management of OME is gathering a detailed history, including the number of episodes of AOM and whether symptoms resolved with appropriate antibiotic therapy. Often a history of RAOM overlaps with persistent OM. A history of allergic rhinitis, GERD, and the presence of symptoms of Eustachian tube dysfunction is helpful to obtain. OME can be readily diagnosed with pneumatic otoscopy. The diagnosis is often confirmed with tympanometry. Physical examination findings that suggest nasal obstruction due to either allergic rhinitis or adenoid hypertrophy prompt additional workup. In cases of chronic nasal obstruction, recurrent rhinosinusitis, or chronic unilateral OME, a flexible nasopharyngoscopy is indicated to rule out adenoid hypertrophy causing obstruction. The International Consensus on the Management of Otitis Media with Effusion in Children recommended using flexible nasopharyngoscopy in areas of the world with a high prevalence of human immunodeficiency virus, which is associated with an increased risk of nasopharyngeal anomalies, including lymphoma.[22]

There are 2 main risk factors for OME with possible direct medical implications, GERD and allergic rhinitis. Although GERD has been associated with OME and pepsin and *Helicobacter pylori* have been isolated from MEEs, the relative prevalence is not high enough to be a major cause of OME. Furthermore, no causation has been established, and there is no definitive evidence that treating GERD will improve or resolve OME. Assessment for GERD is only recommended if there are clinical symptoms, such as epigastric pain, recurrent laryngitis, or sinusitis.[4,22]

Several studies have demonstrated an association between allergic rhinitis and OME.[41–43] Assessment for allergic rhinitis is appropriate if the patient exhibits symptoms such as chronic rhinitis, enlarged inferior turbinate, asthma, or allergies. An allergy contribution to OME should be entertained even for mild symptoms in areas where air quality is poor and there are pollution concerns. Despite proof of an association between OME and allergic rhinitis, there is no convincing evidence that directly treating allergy affects OME outcomes.[22,44]

Observation

For the first time in 2013, national guidelines on the management of OME were published and the indications for TTP emphasized an observation strategy for at least 3 months, especially because MEE after an episode of AOM may eventually clear, avoiding the need for TTP. Serial examinations with possibly a tympanogram, in combination with audiometric testing that shows a hearing loss, allows for an observation strategy. An audiogram is the only formal test routinely required for COME. Half of children will present with a hearing loss of 20 dB or greater. A hearing loss greater than 50 dB is seldom due to OME alone. The 2013 Guidelines recommend an audiogram before ear tube placement, both to determine the need for the procedure based on the established criteria, as well as to determine if there may be a component of sensorineural hearing loss contributing to the loss.[22,36]

Medical treatment

Although several medical therapies have been reported in the treatment of OME, only autoinflation shows some long-term promise at treating the Eustachian tube dysfunction that contributes to OME. Even though treatment with decongestants and antihistamines may help improve concurrent nasal congestion symptoms, treatment of OME does not show any benefit, and these medications can have side effects. Mucolytics may have some short-term efficacy, with one study in particular showing a decrease in the number of patients who met the criteria to have ear tubes placed.[22,45] One review studied the efficacy of continuous antibiotic treatment ranging from 10 days to 6 months and reported no effect of the antibiotic therapy on hearing outcomes, the rate of ear tube insertion, or progression of language development.[22,46] Both oral and nasal steroids have been used in the treatment of OME in an attempt to decrease inflammatory factors in Eustachian tube function and middle ear disease. Multiple studies show no improvement of long-term OME clinical symptoms.[47,48] Oral steroids may have a slight short-term improvement of the OME but the side effects of systemic steroid administration outweigh any short-term benefits. The 2013 Guidelines recommended no steroid treatment.[36]

Surgical treatment

The mainstay of surgical management of OME is the placement of bilateral tympanostomy tubes. The indication for TTP in children with OME is the persistence of MEE longer than 3 months and with at least a 25 dB hearing loss. TTP should also be considered particularly if children exhibit symptoms or sequelae of OME, including vestibular symptoms, poor school performance, behavioral problems, recurrent complaints of ear discomfort, or a perceived decrease in the patient's quality of life.[37] Adjuvant adenoidectomy has been shown to increase the efficacy of OME surgery and can bestow long-lasting beneficial clinical effect for at least 2 years.[49,50] A large prospective study concluded that adjuvant adenoidectomy reduced the risk of OME recurrence requiring subsequent sets of ear tubes, especially in children older than 4 years.[51] Most clinical practice guidelines recommend an adenoidectomy in children with OME older than 4 years and recommend consideration of an adenoidectomy in children with symptomatic adenoid hypertrophy accompanying the OME.[22]

TYMPANOSTOMY TUBES

Once the criteria for ear tube placement have been met and the shared decision to place tubes has been made, several choices of ear tubes exist, depending on the desired material, size, and shape. These factors may determine the tube's propensity to form biofilms and the duration that the tube typically remains in place. The most common short-term tubes that can expect to extrude between 6 months and 12 months after placement are the Shepard tube (made with fluoroplastic or titanium) and the type 1 Paparella tube. Armstrong grommet tubes are fluoroplastic and typically last approximately 14 months and are considered an intermediate stay tube. Silicon T-tubes last for at least 2 years and are considered long-term tubes. They often need to be removed, but because of the silicon material, they can safely be removed in the clinic setting (**Fig. 3**).[36] Compared with short-term tubes, T-tubes have been shown to increase the relative risk of perforation by 3.5 and increase the relative risk of cholesteatoma by 2.6.[52] The decision on which tube should be placed depends on the patient's history, including the presence of comorbidities, such as cleft palate or craniofacial anomalies. The need for multiple sets of ear tubes also prompts shared decision-making discussions about placing T-tubes for the third or subsequent set of ear tubes.

In an effort to reduce the incidence of tube blockage in the immediate postoperative period and to avoid early postoperative otorrhea episodes, particularly when intraoperative findings include MEE, ototopical drops are often used at the time of TTP and for a short postoperative course of ototopical drops.[53,54] The duration of this course of drops is variable, but the type of drops should be those approved by Food and Drug Administration for use in patients with tympanostomy tubes, such as ofloxacin and ciprofloxacin with dexamethasone. Children are typically seen a few weeks after placement of their tympanostomy tubes to confirm appropriate ear

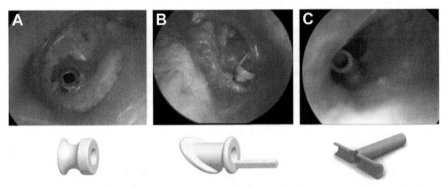

Fig. 3. An example of common types of ear tubes. Each tube is shown individually (bottom) and in position with a view of the tympanic membrane (top). (*A*) Shepard grommets. (*B*) Armstrong grommets. (*C*): T-tubes. (*Adapted from* Simon F, Haggard M, Rosenfeld RM, et. al. International consensus (ICON) on management of otitis media with effusion in children. Eur Ann Otorhinolaryngol Head Neck Dis 2018 Feb;135(1S):S33-S39.)

tube position and to obtain an audiogram, in hopes of documenting normal hearing. Children are usually evaluated every 6 months to document the ear tube position and patency until they ultimately extrude.

Complications and Sequelae of Tympanostomy Tubes

Otorrhea is a common, at times challenging, problem in children with tympanostomy tubes. It is the most frequent complication of TTP, with an incidence as high as 50% of children with tubes reported.[55] Otorrhea is not prevented by observing water precautions but, more likely, occurs when nasal secretions reach the middle ear during a URI through a dysfunctional Eustachian tube.[56,57] The most common bacterial isolate is *Pseudomonas aeruginosa,* which has limited oral antibiotic treatment options for children. The benefit of having tubes in place during an episode of otorrhea is the ability to deliver a much higher concentration of medication directly to the ear. For topical therapy, the Minimum Inhibitory Concentration is irrelevant because this mechanism of delivery achieves a local concentration up to several thousand times higher than that achieved in serum after oral antibiotics.[37] Even if the bacterial isolate is methicillin-resistant *Staphylococcus aureus,* the role of quinolone ototopical medications is extremely important. Oral antibiotics are generally not recommended. Frequent visits to the outpatient clinic may be necessary to suction before administering drops to assure that the drops are being adequately delivered to the middle ear. Cultures of the otorrhea are generally not helpful unless there is refractory drainage despite appropriate aural toilet and adequate treatment with ototopical medications. In these rarer cases, a culture may grow a species of fungus that would prompt a change in the ototopical medication to clotrimazole drops. As a rule of thumb for children with recurrent or persistent tympanostomy tube otorrhea (TTO), 50% of children will recover within 3 to 4 days of ear drops, 90% will recover within 7 days of drops, and 95% will recover within 14 days of ear drops.[37] If the otorrhea persists beyond 2 weeks, additional investigation is conducted into the underlying cause of the otorrhea, based on the laterality and the temporal pattern. If the drainage is unilateral, the underlying cause is more likely to involve local, ear-specific factors such as biofilm formation or granulation tissue. Bilateral TTO suggests a systemic cause. In particular, lack of a "dry period" suggests a chronic underlying condition.[5] Adenoid disease, either chronic infection or hypertrophy, may contribute to recurrent or chronic otorrhea and may benefit from consideration of an adenoidectomy.

Biofilm formation has been shown to contribute to TTO episodes. One study that randomized the type of tube in each ear found that patients with silicone tubes had a longer time to first otorrhea episode.[58] In an in vitro study, Joe and Seo used a Nitinol (nickel–titanium) tympanostomy tube that was smooth with minimized surface area, which was coated with titanium oxide (TiO_2) that formed an oxide layer on the metallic target. Titanium oxide exhibited antibacterial activity and inhibited biofilm formation via a mechanism involving the production of reactive oxygen species.[59] Specific locations on the ear tubes are more susceptible to biofilm formation, specifically in the perpendicular junction between the body and the flanges as well as around the rims of the tube. These zones are potential future target areas in the design or antibiofilm coating materials that may prevent TTO.[60] Targeting the specific DNAB-II biofilm protein could lead to collapse of the biofilm structure. Antibiotic ear drops are the first-line treatment, and a combination of antibiotic and steroid drop seems to be more effective at causing the structural collapse of the biofilm.[61]

Other, less common TM sequelae after tympanostomy tube extrusion include tympanosclerosis, areas of atrophy (most commonly the pars flaccida), and retraction pockets. A metaanalysis estimated the incidence of tympanosclerosis as 32%, focal atrophy as 25%, and of retraction pocket as 3.1%. The type of tube that was placed had no significant impact on these rates.[52] Cayé-Thomasen and colleagues followed 168 subjects for 25 years after myringotomy in the left ear and TTP in the right ear for COME. Myringosclerosis and late atrophy of the TM were more prevalent in the ear with the TTP. The prevalence of TM retraction decreased over the course of the study and the prevalence of myringosclerosis remained unchanged in the ear tube ear and increased in the ears with myringotomy only.[62]

The incidence of persistent TM perforation after ear tube extrusion depends on the type of tube placed. Short-term tubes have an estimated incidence of 2.2% and long-term tubes of 16.6%.[52] Perforations after ear tubes are typically small and therefore, hearing loss, if present, is very mild. They can be easily managed with a myringoplasty using a variety of materials, typically gelfoam or a fat graft. Myringoplasty is more successful if Eustachian tube function is good, otherwise there is a risk of persistent perforation or MEE formation.

The combined incidence of cholesteatoma formation after ear tubes is 0.7% and is slightly higher for long-term tubes. Although an ear tube may actually be placed to reverse a retraction pocket or prevent a cholesteatoma, cholesteatoma may result from tube placement, with ingrowth or transplantation of keratinized epithelium into the middle ear around a tympanostomy tube. An intratympanic cholesteatoma may develop after manipulation of the TM. Children should be monitored carefully at intervals while tubes are in place and after their extrusion for cholesteatoma formation.[5]

A tube may extrude prematurely, typically during or after an infection in the middle ear with otorrhea that "pushes" the tube into the external ear canal. Although rare (3.9% in one study), if the TM is thickened due to inflammation or atrophic, early extrusion is more likely.[52]

Sometimes the lumen of the tympanostomy tube can get blocked by granulation tissue, dry blood, or cerumen. The incidence of plugging of an ear tube is 6.9%.[52] Typically a course of ototopical drops for at least 10 days is a good first step to attempt to unblock the tube. In the outpatient clinic, an instrument such as a pick or small suction can sometimes successfully unblock the tube. If the tube cannot be unblocked but the middle ear is healthy with no MEE, the tube can be left in place until it extrudes. If an MEE develops or recurrent infections occur, the tube may need to be replaced.[5]

Rarely, a tube or tubes need to be removed in the operating room with a myringoplasty procedure performed. Indications for removing a tympanostomy tube include the following: (1) one tube is retained, whereas the other tube has extruded with a healthy middle ear for at least 1 year and the patient is older than 5 years, (2) bilateral retained tubes in an older child with normal Eustachian tube function, (3) chronic or recurrent otorrhea resistant to medical therapy, and (4) the tympanostomy tube is imbedded in granulation tissue and the tube is blocked.[5] In a case-control study by Huestis and colleagues, retained tubes that went on to require removal in the operating room were placed more often for RAOM as the indication rather than COME.[63]

The 2013 Clinical Practice Guideline also recommended that clinicians not encourage routine, prophylactic water precautions, such as the use of earplugs or headbands, or the avoidance of swimming or water sports for children with tympanostomy tubes.[36] The most compelling evidence against routine water precautions for tympanostomy tubes comes from a large randomized controlled trial comparing swimming/bathing with ear plugs and without over a 9-month period. Although there were some statistically significant benefits to routine ear plug use, the clinical benefit was trivial: a child would need to wear plugs for 2.8 years, on average, to prevent a single episode of otorrhea.[64]

CLINICS CARE POINTS

- AOM should be treated with oral antibiotics in children younger than 6 months, even if the diagnosis is uncertain or the symptoms are not severe.
- AOM may be observed in children older than 6 months if the diagnosis is uncertain or if the diagnosis is certain but the symptoms are not severe. If symptoms are severe, they should be treated with oral antibiotics.
- Risk factors for the development of RAOM are age, craniofacial anomalies, genetic predisposition, daycare attendance, tobacco smoke exposure, and seasonality of URIs.
- Tympanostomy tubes are recommended for children who have more than 3 AOM infections in 6 months or more than 4 in 12 months with one recent and if the ear examination at the time of the clinic visit is not normal.
- COME is the presence of MEE in one or both ears for 3 months or longer.
- Risk factors for the development of COME are Eustachian tube dysfunction, recurrent infections, and to a lesser degree, allergy, and GERD.
- Tympanostomy tubes are recommended for children who have an MEE in one or both ears for 3 months or longer.
- For children with COME older than 4 years or with chronic nasal obstruction symptoms, adjunctive adenoidectomy may decrease episodes of tympanostomy tube otorrhea and the need for subsequent sets of ear tubes.
- Children with tympanostomy tubes should be closely monitored for complications of ear tubes, including otorrhea, TM perforation, retraction pocket/atrophy of TM, and cholesteatoma even after the tubes extrude.
- Complications of AOM are typically infectious and are most commonly intratemporal but may be intracranial as well. Often a mastoidectomy is required in addition to TTP.
- Complications of OME most commonly involve the corresponding hearing loss such as speech and language delay. Children with persistent MEE may experience episodes of vertigo as part of their clinical course.

DISCLOSURE

The author has nothing to disclose.

REFERENCES

1. Tos M. Epidemiology and natural history of secretory otitis. Am J Otol 1984;5: 459–62.
2. Mandel EM, Doyle WJ, Winther B, et al. The incidence, prevalence and burden of OM in unselected children aged 1-8 years followed by weekly otoscopy through the "common cold" season. Int J Pediatr Otorhinolaryngol 2008;72:491–9.
3. Lieberthal AS, Carroll AE, Chonmaitree T. The diagnosis and management of acute otitis media. Pediatrics 2013;131:e964–99.
4. Rosenfeld RM, Shin JJ, Schwartz SR, et al. Clinical practice guideline: otitis media with effusion (update). Otolaryngol Head Neck Surg 2016;154:S1–41.
5. Casselbrant ML, Mandel EM. Otitis media in the age of antimicrobial resistance. Bailey's Head & Neck surgery otolaryngology. 5th edition. Philadelphia: Wolters Kluwer/Lippincott Williams & Wilkins; 2014. p. 1479–506.
6. Hoffman HJ, Park J, Losonczy KG, et al. Risk factors, treatments, and other conditions associated with frequent ear infections in US children through 2 years of

age: the early childhood longitudinal study – birth cohort (ECLS-B). Presented at 9th International Symposium on Recent Advances in Otitis Media, St. Pete Beach, FL, June 3–7, 2007.

7. Casselbrant ML, Brostoff LM, Cantekin EI, et al. Otitis media with effusion in pre-school children. Laryngoscope 1985;95(4):428–36.

8. Teele DW, Klein JO, Rosner B. Epidemiology of otitis media during the first seven years of life in children in greater Boston: a prospective, cohort study. J Infect Dis 1989;160(1):83–94.

9. Pukander JS, Karma PH. Persistence of middle ear effusion and its risk factors after an acute attack of otitis media with effusion. In: Lim DJ, Bluestone CD, Klein JO, Nelson JD, editors. Recent advances in otitis media. Bal Harbour, Florida: Proceedings of the Fourth International Symposium; June 1-4, 1987.

10. Bluestone CD, Klein JO. Otitis media in infants and children. 4th edition. Hamilton (Ontario): BC Decker Inc.; 2007.

11. Robinson PJ, Lodge S, Jones BM, et al. The effect of palate repair on otitis media with effusion. Plast Reconstr Surg 1992;89(4):640–5.

12. Casselbrant ML, Mandel EM, Fall PA, et al. The heritability of otitis media: a twin and triplet study. JAMA 1999;282(22):2125–30.

13. Daly KA, Brown WM, Segade F, et al. Chronic and recurrent otitis media: a genome scan for susceptibility loci. Am J Hum Genet 2004;75(6):988–97.

14. Heikkinen T, Thint M, Chonmaitree T. Prevalence of various respiroatory viruses in the middle ear during acute otitis media. N Engl J Med 1999;340(4):260–4.

15. Pitkäranta A, Virolainen A, Jero J, et al. Detection of rhinovirus, respiratory syncytial virus, and corona virus infections in acute otitis media by reverse transcriptase polymerase chain reaction. Pediatrics 1998;102(2):291–5.

16. Fiellau-Nikolajsen M. Tympanometry in three-year old children. Type of care as an epidemiological factor in secretory otitis media and tubal dysfunction in unselected populations of three year old children. ORL Otorhinolaryngol Relat Spec 1979;41(4):193–205.

17. Chantry CJ, Howard CR, Auinger P. Full breastfeeding duration and associated decrease in respiratory tract infection in US children. Pediatrics 2006;117(2):425–32.

18. Smith DF, Boss EF. Racial/ethnic and socioeconomic disparities in the prevalence and treatment of otitis media in children in the United States. Laryngoscope 2010;120(11):2306–12.

19. Niemelä M, Pihakari O, Pokka T, et al. Pacifier as a risk factor for acute otitis media: a randomized, controlled trial of parental counseling. Pediatrics 2000;106(3):483–8.

20. Bluestone CD. Eustachian tube: structure, function, role in otitis media. Hamilton (Ontario): BC Decker Inc.; 2005.

21. Maw AR, Bawden R. The long term outcome of secretory otitis media in children and the effects of surgical treatment: a ten year study. Acta Otorhinolaryngol Belg 1994;48:317–24.

22. Simon F, Haggard M, Rosenfeld RM, et al. International consensus (ICON) on management of otitis media with effusion in children. Eur Ann Otorhinolaryngol Head Neck Dis 2018;135(1S):S33–9.

23. Post JC, Preston RA, Aul JJ, et al. Molecular analysis of bacterial pathogens in otitis media with effusion. JAMA 1995;273(20):1598–604.

24. Heikkinen T, Chonmaitree T. Importance of respiratory viruses in acute otitis media. Clin Microbiol Rev 2003;16(2):230–41.

25. Skoner DP, Doyle WJ, Chamovitz AH, et al. Eustachian tube obstruction after intranasal challenge with house dust mite. Arch Otolaryngol 1986;112(8):840–2.

26. Faden H. The microbiologic and immunologic basis for recurrent otitis media in children. Eur J Pediatr 2001;160(7):407–13.

27. Straetemans M, van Heerbeek N, Sanders EA, et al. Immune status and Eustachian tube function in recurrence of otitis media with effusion. Arch Otolaryngol Head Neck Surg 2005;131(9):771–6.

28. Lechien JR, Hans S, Simon F, et al. Association between laryngopharyngeal reflux and otitis media: a systematic review. Otol Neurotol 2021;42(7):e801–14.

29. Wu ZH, Tang Y, Niu X, et al. The relationship between otitis media with effusion and gastroesophageal reflux disease: a meta-analysis. Otol Neurotol 2021; 42(3):e245–53.

30. Fireman B, Black SB, Shinefield HR, et al. Impact of the pneumococcal conjugate vaccine on otitis media. Pediatr Infect Dis J 2003;22(1):10–6.

31. Norhayati MN, Ho JJ, Azman MY. Influenza vaccines for preventing acute otitis media in infants and children. Cochrane Database Syst Rev 2017;10(10): CD010089.

32. American Academy of Pediatrics Subcommittee on Management of Acute Otitis Media. Diagnosis and management of acute otitis media. Pediatrics 2004;113(5): 1451–65.

33. Mattos JL, Colman KL, Casselbrant ML, et al. Intratemporal and intracranial complications of acute otitis media in a pediatric population. Int J Pediatr Otorhinolaryngol 2014;78(12):2161–4.

34. Leach AJ, Morris PS. Antibiotics for the prevention of acute and chronic suppurative otitis media in children. Cochrane Database Syst Rev 2006;(4):CD004401.

35. Marom T, Marchisio P, Tamir SO, et al. Complementary and alternative medicine treatment options for otitis media: a systematic review. Medicine (Baltimore) 2016;95(6):e2695.

36. Rosenfeld RM, Schwartz SR, Pynnonen MA, et al. Clinical Practice Guideline: Tympanostomy Tubes in Children. Otolaryngol Head Neck Surg 2013;149(IS): S1–35.

37. Rosenfeld RM. Tympanostomy tube controversies and issues: state-of-the-art review. Ear Nose Throat J 2020;99(1_suppl):15S–21S.

38. Bluestone CD. Eustachian tube dysfunction: physiology, pathophysiology, and roll of allergy in pathogenesis of otitis media. J Allergy Clin Immunol 1983; 72(3):242–51.

39. Brook I, Shah K, Jackson W. Microbiology of healthy and diseased adenoids. Laryngoscope 2000;110(6):994–9.

40. Coticchia J, Zuliani G, Coleman C, et al. Biofilm surface area in the pediatric nasopharynx: chronic rhinosinusitis vs. obstructive sleep apnea. Arch Otolaryngol Head Neck Surg 2007;133(2):110–4.

41. Luong A, Roland PS. The link between allergic rhinitis and chronic otitis media with effusion in atopic patients. Otolaryngol Clin North Am 2008;41:311–23.

42. Kleinman-Møller E, Chawes BL, Caye-Thomasen P, et al. Allergic rhinitis is associated with otitis media with effusion: a birth cohort study. Clin Exp Allergy 2012; 42(11):1615–20.

43. Kwon C, Lee HY, Kim MG, et al. Allergic diseases in children with otitis media with effusion. Int J Pediatr Otorhinolaryngol 2013;77:158–61.

44. Griffin G, Flynn CA. Antihistamines and/or decongestants for otitis media with effusion (OME) in children. Cochrane Database Syst Rev 2011;(9):Cd003423.

45. Moore RA, Commins D, Bates G, et al. S-carboxymethylcysteine in the treatment of glue ear: quantitative systematic review. BMC Fam Pract 2001;2:3.
46. Venekamp RP, Burton MJ, van Dongen GJ, et al. Antibiotics for otitis media with effusion in children. Cochrane Database Syst Rev 2016;(6):Cd009163.
47. Simpson SA, Lewis R, van der Voort J, et al. Oral or topical nasal steroids for hearing loss associated with otitis media with effusion in children. Cochrane Database Syst Rev 2011;(5):Cd001935.
48. Roditi RE, Rosenfeld RM, Shin JJ. Otitis media with effusion: our national practice. Otolaryngol Head Neck Surg 2017;157(2):171–2.
49. Boonacker CW, Rovers MM, Browning GG, et al. Adenoidectomy with or without grommets for children with otitis media: an individual patient data meta-analysis. Health Technol Assess 2014;18:1–118.
50. van der Aardweg MT, Schilder AG, Herkert E, et al. Adenoidectomy for otitis media in children. Cochrane Database Syst Rev 2010;(1):CD007810.
51. Wang MC, Wang YP, Chu CH, et al. The protective effect of adenoidectomy on pediatric tympanostomy tube re-insertions: a population-based birth cohort study. PLoS One 2014;9:e101175.
52. Kay DJ, Nelson M, Rosenfeld RM. Meta-analysis of tympanostomy tube sequelae. Otolaryngol Head Neck Surg 2001;124:374–80.
53. Elden LM, Marsh RR. Survey of pediatric otolaryngologists: clinical practice trends used to prevent and treat blocked ventilation ear tubes in children. Int J Pediatr Otorhinolaryngol 2006;70(9):1533–8.
54. Giles W, Dohar J, Iverson K, et al. Ciprofloxacin/dexamethasone drops decrease the incidence of physician and patient outcomes of otorrhea after tube placement. Int J Pediatr Otorhinolaryngol 2007;71(5):747–56.
55. Vlastarakos PV, Nikolopoulos TP, Korres S, et al. Grommets in otitis media with effusion: the most frequent operation in children. But is it associated with significant complications? Eur J Pediatr 2007;166:385–91.
56. Pringle MB. Grommets, swimming and otorrhea–a review. J Laryngol Otol 1993; 107:190–4.
57. Moualed D, Masterson L, Kumar S, et al. Water precautions for prevention of infection in children with ventilation tubes (grommets). Cochrane Database Syst Rev 2016;(1):Cd010375.
58. Knutsson J, Priwin C, Hessen-Soderman AC, et al. A randomized study of four different types of tympanostomy ventilation tubes—full-term follow-up. Int J Pediatr Otorhinolaryngol 2018;107:140–4.
59. Joe H, Seo YJ. A newly designed tympanostomy stent with TiO2 coating to reduce Pseudomonas aeruginosa biofilm formation. J Biomater Appl 2018; 33(4):599–605.
60. Marom T, Habashi N, Cohen R, et al. Role of biofilms in post-tympanostomy tube otorrhea. Ear Nose Throat J 2020;99(1_suppl):22S–9S.
61. van Dongen TMA, Damoiseaux RAMJ, Schilder AGM. Tympanostomy tube otorrhea in children: prevention and treatment. Curr Opin Otolaryngol Head Neck Surg 2018;26(6):437–40.
62. Cayé-Thomasen P, Stangerup SE, Jørgensen G, et al. Myringotomy versus ventilation tubes in secretory otitis media: eardrum pathology, hearing, and eustachian tube function 25 years after treatment. Otol Neurotol 2008;29(5):649–57.
63. Huestis MJ, Shehan JN, Levi JR. Factors associated with retained tympanostomy tubes a case-controlled study. Int J Pediatr Otorhinolaryngol 2020;138:110317.
64. Goldstein NA, Mandel EM, Kurs-Lasky M, et al. Water precautions and tympanostomy tubes: a randomized, controlled trial. Laryngoscope 2005;115(2):324–30.

Congenital Sensorineural Hearing Loss

Samantha Shave, BS[a], Christina Botti, MS[b], Kelvin Kwong, MD[a],*

KEYWORDS

- Pediatric hearing loss • Sensorineural hearing loss • Congenital hearing loss
- Children • Diagnosis • Treatment • Review

KEY POINTS

- Being the most common sensory deficit, congenital sensorineural hearing loss has diverse causes.
- Advancement in genomic sequencing technology allows us to better understand the genetic contribution to congenital hearing loss. Comprehensive genetic evaluation has become the cornerstone of the clinical workup of congenital hearing loss.
- Early diagnosis and intervention are key to improving the developmental outcomes of children with congenital sensorineural hearing loss.
- Indications and candidacy of hearing amplification technologies, such as bone conduction hearing device, cochlear implant, and auditory brainstem implant have been expanded, supported by the evidence of current research.

INTRODUCTION

Congenital hearing loss can be defined as hearing loss present at birth and is due to an impairment in the conduction and/or conversion of sound into electrical nerve impulses.[1] Permanent congenital hearing loss is the most common sensory deficit, with a prevalence of 1.2 to 1.7 individuals per 1000 live births in the United States[2]; 20% to 30% of those children have profound hearing loss. Hearing loss can be characterized as conductive—deficits in the outer or middle ear—or sensorineural—impairment in the inner ear, auditory nerve, or central auditory pathway.[1] Sensorineural congenital hearing loss is caused by inner ear damage or issues with the nerve pathways that transmit sound from the inner ear to the auditory cortex in the brain.

Financial Disclosures: None.
Conflicts of Interest: None.
[a] Department of Otolaryngology–Head & Neck Surgery, Division of Pediatric Otolaryngology, Rutgers Robert Wood Johnson Medical School, 10 Plum Street, 8th Floor, New Brunswick, NJ 08901, USA; [b] Department of Pediatrics, Division of Medical Genetics, Rutgers Robert Wood Johnson Medical School, 10 Plum Street, 8th Floor, New Brunswick, NJ 08901, USA
* Corresponding author.
E-mail address: kelvin.kwong@rutgers.edu

Pediatr Clin N Am 69 (2022) 221–234
https://doi.org/10.1016/j.pcl.2021.12.006
0031-3955/22/© 2022 Elsevier Inc. All rights reserved.

Sensorineural congenital hearing loss can be further classified into syndromic and nonsyndromic depending on whether there are malformations or medical conditions involving other organ systems associated with hearing loss. Treatment of congenital hearing loss will depend on the type and cause of the condition.

Sensorineural hearing loss is classified by a variety of different characteristics. Hearing loss can be unilateral or bilateral, and the degree of hearing impairment can range from a difficulty with understanding soft speech (mild) to an inability to hear loud noises (profound). Hearing loss may also be stable or progress over time. A particular type of sensorineural hearing loss shows a distinctive mild to moderate U-shaped or "cookie-bite" dip in hearing threshold across midfrequency, whereas the high and low frequencies are preserved. This pattern of hearing loss is traditionally thought to have a hereditary and familial association. However, a recent study using exome sequencing data showed that more than 80% of subjects with a cookie-bite audiogram did not carry a genetic variant in known hearing loss gene.[3] This is just one of many examples how expanded genetic information improves our understanding of hearing loss.

Detection of congenital hearing loss is critical, considering that early diagnosis and medical intervention have been shown to lead to improved developmental outcomes.[4] The American Academy of Pediatrics' Joint Committee on Infant Hearing proposed the 1-3-6 guidelines for early hearing detection and intervention.[5] To maximize the outcomes for infants with significant hearing impairment, the hearing of all infants should be screened at no later than 1 month of age. Those who do not pass screening should have a comprehensive audiologic evaluation no later than 3 months of age. Infants with confirmed hearing loss should receive appropriate intervention at no later than 6 months of age from health care and education professionals.[5] Without intervention and treatment, hearing loss can have a significant impact on speech, language, education, and other developmental cognitive skills.[6] Despite such effort in early detection and intervention, due to the progressive nature of some subtypes of congenital hearing loss, early infant screenings can often miss patients with this sensory deficit; this makes repeat screenings at regular intervals particularly critical for at-risk neonates.

Although congenital hearing loss can be conductive in nature or related to auditory neuropathy spectrum disorder, the majority is sensorineural hearing loss. This review focuses on congenital sensorineural hearing loss in the pediatric population and its epidemiology, causes, risk factors, inheritance, and treatments. In addition, we emphasize clinical decision-making strategies, as well as management and treatment of hereditary sensorineural hearing loss. By developing a greater understanding of the characterization, prevalence, current diagnostics, available genetic testing, and the underlying mechanisms of sensorineural hearing loss, we can promote improvements in clinical decision making, prognosis, and treatment of patients with sensorineural hearing impairment.

CAUSE OF CONGENITAL HEARING LOSS

Conventionally, about 50% of congenital hearing loss was known to be associated with genetic causes, whereas about 25% were considered idiopathic, suggesting significant gaps of knowledge in this particular area. With ongoing advancement in genetic knowledge, it has been reported, in developed countries, that up to 80% of congenital hearing loss is due to genetic causes with the remaining 20% secondary to environmental or acquired causes[7] **(Fig. 1)**. Acquired hearing loss in children commonly results from either prenatal "TORCH" infection, namely, toxoplasmosis, syphilis, rubella, cytomegalovirus, and herpes, or postnatal bacterial meningitis

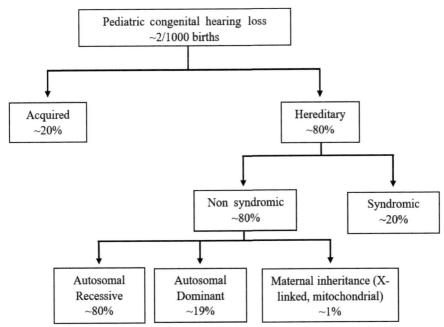

Fig. 1. Causes of prelingual hearing loss in developed countries. Adapted with permission from "Hereditary Hearing Loss and Deafness Overview" by Shearer AE, Hildebrand MS, Smith RJH[7]

caused by various organisms.[8] Genetically related or hereditary hearing loss can be subdivided into syndromic (20%) or nonsyndromic (80%) form (see **Fig. 1**). Although syndromic hearing loss can involve malformations of multiple other organ systems besides the ear, an early diagnosis may not be apparent as the classic signs and symptoms may manifest later in life. Nonsyndromic sensorineural hearing loss is heterogeneous. Autosomal recessive nonsyndromic hearing loss accounts for 80% of genetic cases, and autosomal dominant nonsyndromic hearing loss accounts for about 15% to 20% of cases. Autosomal dominant nonsyndromic hearing loss is often progressive and has a later age of onset. X-linked or maternal mitochondrial DNA-related modes of inheritance are rare, and each accounts for approximately 1% of nonsyndromic hearing loss.[9,10]

Heterogeneity of Hereditary Hearing Loss

The heterogeneous nature of hereditary hearing loss makes the elucidation of the underlying causes challenging. More than 400 genetic syndromes are associated with hearing loss, and more than 110 gene mutations that are associated with nonsyndromic hearing loss have been identified.[7] With the advent of whole-genome sequencing (WGS), the number of syndromes and genes associated with hearing loss continues to grow. Genes associated with hereditary hearing loss encode a wide variety of proteins important for the auditory pathway development and functions, such as transcription factors, structural proteins, gap junction proteins, and ion channels.[7] The mode of inheritance for syndromic hearing loss can be autosomal dominant (Waardenburg syndrome, branchio-oto-renal syndrome, neurofibromatosis type 2 [NF2]), autosomal recessive (Stickler syndrome, Usher syndrome, Mohr-Tranebjaerg syndrome), or X-linked (80% of Alport, syndrome). Most hereditary hearing loss (80%) is nonsyndromic, which is characterized by tremendous genetic variability and heterogeneity suggested by more than 6000 causative variants in more than 110 genes.[7] Almost 80% of nonsyndromic hearing loss is inherited in an autosomal recessive pattern. In addition, in most cases, nonsyndromic hearing loss is due to a single genetic factor.[11] Accounting for an estimated 50% of all autosomal recessive nonsyndromic hearing loss in the Caucasian European and US population, DFNB1 locus includes GJB2 and GJB6 genes that encode the gap junction protein, connexin 26 and 30, respectively, functionally involved in maintaining K^+ homeostasis in the inner ear.[12–14] GJB2-related hearing loss is sensorineural, usually present at birth, typically bilateral and nonprogressive, and can range from mild to profound in severity. However, progressive or later-onset hearing loss—with infants passing their newborn hearing screen—have also been described, particularly in association with nontruncating mutations.[15–18]

More than 25 genes have been associated with autosomal dominant nonsyndromic hearing loss.[7] With respect to the clinical importance in pediatric congenital hearing loss, most of autosomal dominant genes cause postlingual hearing loss except for GJB2 and GJB6 found in DFNA3 locus, TECTA in DFNA8/12 locus, SIX1 in DFNA23, and WFS1 in DFNA 6/14/38 locus. Nonsyndromic mitochondrial hearing loss is associated with genes encoding the mitochondrial 12S ribosomal RNA (MTRNR1) and mitochondrial transfer RNA (MT-TS1). MTRNR1 mutation is of particular importance in pediatric patients with significant history of neonatal intensive care unit (NICU) stay because the gene is associated with predisposition to ototoxicity from aminoglycoside, which is a commonly used antimicrobial medication in the NICU setting.

RISK FACTORS OTHER THAN GENETIC CAUSE

Despite the high frequency of genetic involvement in congenital hearing loss overall, approximately 1.43% of cases have a positive family history of hearing loss.[1] In addition to genetic mutations, hearing loss can also result from environmental factors or exposures. Environmental causes of hearing loss include certain medications, specific infections before or after birth, and exposure to loud noise over an extended period. Evidence suggests that infectious factors including rubella, cytomegalovirus, and acquired immunodeficiency syndrome can be potential nongenetic causes of nonsyndromic sensorineural hearing loss.[19] The development of the inner ear takes place during the first trimester of pregnancy, and therefore, disturbances at this stage, whether due to genetic mutations or environmental disturbances, can result in hearing loss.[20] Owing to the possibility and prevalence of infectious agents causing acquired nonsyndromic sensorineural hearing loss, testing for these factors is critical.[9,21] Congenital rubella is now a less frequent cause of hearing loss as a result of immunization.[22,23]

Congenital CMV (cCMV) infection is the most common cause of nonhereditary hearing loss among children in the United States. According to the Centers for Disease Control and Prevention (CDC), approximately 1 in 200 babies are born with cCMV and 1 of 5 of those babies will experience symptoms or long-term health problems, including hearing loss. In the first and second trimesters of pregnancy, the risk of transmission is 30% to 40%, and increases to 40% to 70% in the third trimester.[24] Transmission of CMV from the mother to the child can occur transplancentally, during delivery, and through breast milk; however, transmission via delivery and breast milk are not associated with central nervous system complications.[25] Of the infants born with cCMV infection each year, 85% to 90% are asymptomatic at birth; however, 10% to 15% of these infants will develop sensorineural hearing loss.[21] cCMV-associated hearing loss can present in early childhood, and can be unilateral or bilateral, but is more commonly unilateral and progressive. In addition, approximately 33% to 50% of sensorineural hearing loss caused by cCMV is late onset and may remain undetected even in children who undergo newborn hearing screening and receive a thorough physical examination. Therefore, cCMV can be considered a major cause of both congenital and delayed-onset sensorineural hearing loss, making early identification of cCMV infection important to both the prognosis and treatment of children with hearing impairment.[26–30]

EVALUATION STRATEGY
General Considerations

Owing to the diversity of causes and degrees of pediatric congenital hearing loss, clinical judgment is key during the clinical evaluation process. Diagrammatic overview of the general approach to clinical evaluation of pediatric congenital hearing loss is shown in **Fig. 2**. Actual clinical decisions may vary, depending on individual patient's presentation and history. All newborns and infants who fail newborn hearing screen should undergo diagnostic testing for auditory brainstem response or auditory steady state response to confirm the hearing loss. Once the hearing loss is confirmed, the child should proceed with a comprehensive medical evaluation, which includes the following important components: (1) a pertinent perinatal history including prenatal exposure to maternal infections (eg, CMV, rubella, syphilis), drugs and medications (eg, thalidomide, retinoic acid), prematurity, low birth weight, hyperbilirubinemia, ototoxic medication (eg, aminoglycoside), and postnatal history of head trauma and bacterial meningitis; (2) a detailed family history that identifies first- and second-degree relatives with hearing loss and commonly associated features such as renal anomaly and cardiac issues; and (3) a physical examination focusing on identifying

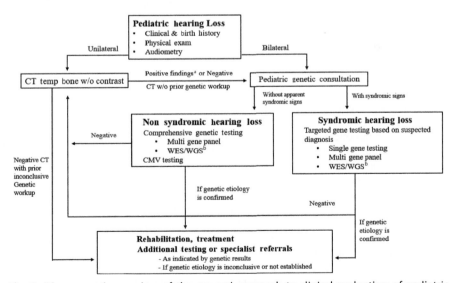

Fig. 2. Diagrammatic overview of the general approach to clinical evaluation of pediatric congenital hearing loss. CT, computed tomography; temp, temporal; w/o, without; WES, whole-exome sequencing. [a]Enlarged vestibular aqueduct, Michel deformity, incomplete cochlear partition, common cavity, etc. [b]Whole-exome sequencing/whole-genome sequencing.

unusual facial features, branchial cleft and ear anomaly, skin or hair pigmentation, and neurologic findings.

Hearing Loss Characteristics

Whether the hearing loss is bilateral or unilateral has a significant implication on the first step of the evaluation process. Precaido and colleagues[31] studied 150 children with idiopathic pediatric sensorineural hearing loss in a prospective prevalence study, showing that none of the patients with unilateral sensorineural hearing loss had positive GJB2 screen. Meanwhile, the diagnostic yield of computed tomographic (CT) temporal bone scan was highest among this group of children compared with those with bilateral sensorineural hearing loss, regardless of the severity of hearing loss.[31] These data suggest that imaging studies are the most appropriate initial workup for children with unilateral sensorineural hearing loss (see **Fig. 2**). Both CT and MRI are used in the evaluation of pediatric hearing loss with advantages and disadvantages in each modality. CT scan of temporal bone is relatively less costly, is more time efficient, and can be done without sedation in most cases. With a small dose of ionizing radiation, CT can provide excellent bony details of the inner ear that captures various cochlear anomalies, the most common being enlarged vestibular aqueduct. Although MRI is more expensive and usually requires sedation due to the duration of image acquisition, it does provide details about the cochlear nerve that CT cannot, enabling the proper diagnosis of cochlear hypoplasia or aplasia. The positive results of imaging studies provide important information to tailor the subsequent genetic workup. For example, patients with enlarged vestibular aqueduct are associated with mutation of the SLC26A4 gene found in Pendred syndrome.

At present, there is no general consensus over the choice of imaging modality or the timing of obtaining imaging studies.[32] In a consensus statement on pediatric hearing loss from the International Pediatric Otolaryngology Group (IPOG), there was 100% consensus that children who are cochlear implant candidates with profound hearing loss may benefit from CT or MRI to assess for cochlear dysplasias and cochlear nerve aplasia. Moreover, IPOG expressed a majority opinion that temporal bone imaging can be postponed to a later age during the neonatal period unless indicated for other reasons, such as neurologic workup that requires MRI of the brain.[33]

Importance of Genetic Evaluation and Consultation

For patients presenting with bilateral pediatric hearing loss, a genetic consultation would be the appropriate first step. Patients with unilateral hearing loss may also benefit from a genetic evaluation after the initial imaging workup (see **Fig. 2**). A clinical genetics evaluation including genetic counseling is important for children and families with sensorineural hearing loss. There are several benefits to the establishment of a genetic cause including providing etiologic information, identifying and possibly allying concerns about comorbidities that may require additional referrals, and planning for future concerns, which may include surgery or educational modifications, ability to offer recurrence risks, and the establishment of psychological well-being.[34] In some cases, guidance can be provided to avoid certain exposures for at-risk family members to mitigate ototoxicity.[35]

When an individual is referred for genetic consultation, several factors are included in determining the most appropriate test. For individuals with hearing loss, a focused medical and birth history as well as a three-generation pedigree will need to be obtained. A physical examination focusing on dysmorphic features is performed. For those individuals who do not seem to have any signs of syndromic hearing loss, CMV testing is coordinated (see **Fig. 2**). The diagnosis of cCMV-related hearing loss can be challenging to make, because it is characterized by variable hearing loss severity ranging from asymptomatic to severe, as well as bilateral, asymmetric, or unilateral sensorineural hearing loss.[36] To ascertain cCMV as the cause for hearing loss in newborns, polymerase chain reaction (PCR) testing for CMV DNA in the urine, saliva (preferred specimens), blood, or dried blood spot taken at birth should be done within 3 weeks of birth, given the ubiquity of the virus in the environment.[9] With high sensitivity and specificity, PCR test is considerably quicker than the traditional CMV culture technique, which can take up to 4 to 5 days for the test to turnaround. In children older than 3 weeks, a negative CMV Ig titer can rule out CMV as the cause for congenital hearing loss. However, a positive CMV Ig titer cannot confirm that the hearing loss is due to cCMV infection as the patients may be exposed to CMV postnatally. While not widely available in commerical laboratory, PCR testing for CMV DNA in neonatal dried blood spot is available in either the CDC laboratory or two university-affliated laboratories at the University of Utah and the University of Minnesota. In the past, single-gene sequencing such as GJB2 was the initial step in establishing a diagnosis. However, advances in genetic sequencing technology allow the development of a new generation of genetic tests that are rapidly replacing this testing modality.

Advances in Genetic Testing

Next-generation sequencing (NGS), also known as massively parallel sequencing, is a modern sequencing technology that can process multiple DNA sequences in parallel, providing orders of magnitude of higher data throughput at a much lower cost when compared with conventional Sanger sequencing method. NGS uses disease-targeted exon capture, whole exome sequencing (WES), or WGS strategies.[37,38] The ability to look at multiple genes causing a single disorder (ie, genetic heterogeneity) is a significant advantage to this technology. These tests are an excellent way to assess many genes associated with a specific condition or more globally assessing for hearing loss. A limitation to testing using NGS is that it will sequence only genes that are known to be associated with hearing loss or a particular syndrome. WES does not solely rely on a list of genes involved in a disease process but rather evaluates all exons in the genome for variations; this would allow for the identification of variants in known hearing loss genes as well as in genes that may have yet to be identified to be associated with hearing loss. WGS evaluates the genome, which has the potential to identify changes outside of the exons that may be related to hearing loss.

When counseling families or individuals about genetic testing options it is important to discuss limitations of testing as well. Although NGS continues to improve as a technology, a clinician must always assess if the test has appropriate gene coverage, sensitivity, and the types of variants that are detected. As opposed to WGS, not all regions are evaluated when using NGS or WES, because large deletions and duplications in addition to copy number or structural variants may not be detected.

An important counseling consideration when offering WES or WGS is that although the ability to detect a larger variety of hearing loss-related changes increases, so will the difficulty with interpretation. The more genes analyzed the more variants there are likely to be identified. Causally linking the variants to new genes associated with hearing loss or genetic susceptibility to hearing loss can be difficult and time consuming. Potential outcomes of testing include pathogenic, likely pathogenic, variant of uncertain significance, likely benign, and benign. Pretest counseling is imperative to help decrease confusion later. Variants of uncertain significance cause the most anxiety. These are variants in which the association with disease risk is unclear. Additional testing may be required, which may include testing of other family members. These results can be confusing to clinicians, not to mention families.

For individuals with findings suggestive of a syndrome genetic cause, there are several options available (see **Fig. 2**). Should a syndrome have a single gene causing the disease, single-gene testing can be ordered. Should multiple genes be known to cause a particular condition, for example, Waardenburg syndrome, an NGS multigene panel can be considered. If those are nondiagnostic, microarray, WES, or WGS can then be considered. Targeted secondary tests should be included in the evaluation depending on the syndrome being considered. Appropriate referrals should be made depending on associated manifestations specific to the syndrome being considered.

As with all genetic testing, pretest genetic counseling should be provided, and with the patient's informed consent, genetic testing can proceed. If genetic testing fails to reveal an underlying cause and there is no prior imaging workup done, patients will benefit from having dedicated CT temporal bone imaging to look for potential inner ear anomalies (see **Fig. 2**). If the results of both genetic and imaging workups are negative, the congenital hearing loss is considered idiopathic, which accounts for up to 25% to 30% of cases undergoing the workup.[39] Ophthalmology consultation and electrocardiography together with renal ultrasonography are recommended to evaluate for potential significant morbidities associated with hearing loss. Despite being uncommon (ie, <1%), prolonged QT interval-associated Jervell and Lange-Nielsen syndrome can be potentially life threatening if not recognized and left untreated. Ophthalmologic findings, predominantly unrecognized refractive errors as well as strabismus and amblyopia, are relatively common in patients with congenital hearing loss.[40] It is particularly important to identify and treat visual issues in hearing-impaired children who are already at risk of developing speech delays. Periodic follow-up is recommended every 2 to 3 years. This recommendation is due to a few reasons including syndrome presentation varying by age. Some symptoms may not manifest in young children and become more evident with time. Another reason is that with time, our understanding of our genes increases so that more genes can either be included on panels or be more easily interpreted. New genetic tests are developed in time so that other technologies may be used to interrogate the genetic information.

TREATMENT OPTIONS
Conventional Hearing Amplification

One of the main goals of treatment of pediatric hearing loss is to promote speech and language development. Access to sound (ie, satisfactory sound amplification) is the cornerstone of a successful treatment of children with significant hearing loss. Age at fitting amplification has the largest influence of speech development and spoken language outcome.[41] Other factors affecting the intervention outcome include the degree of hearing loss, hours of amplification usage, intensity of oral education, and parental interaction. It is well documented that even mild hearing loss can be associated with significant learning disadvantages and speech development delays leading to poor academic performance. For children with bilateral hearing loss, there are several advantages of using bilateral amplification including improved sound localization, better speech discrimination in noise, and prevention of auditory deprivation of the unaided ear. Based on the American Academy of Audiology Clinical Practice Guidelines on Pediatric Amplification, behind-the-ear (BTE) hearing aid is the recommended style of choice.[42] As children's outer ears are constantly growing until puberty, refitting the ear mold of BTE hearing aid is relatively inexpensive, compared with the in-the-ear style. BTE hearing aid provides appropriate coupling to a variety of assistive listening devices used in educational and social settings (eg, FM system).

Cochlear Implantation

Cochlear implant takes the amplification to the next level that conventional hearing aids are not able to achieve due to the limitation of audio feedback loop gain between the microphone and the speaker. Cochlear implant bypasses the defective outer hair cells by providing direct electrical stimulation to the spiral ganglion cells of the auditory nerve. Cochlear implants have been approved by the US Food and Drug Administration (FDA) for use in pediatric population since 1990. As of December 2019, approximately 736,900 registered devices have been implanted worldwide. In the United States, roughly 118,100 devices have been implanted in adults and 65,000 in children based on the estimate provided by US FDA.[43] Cochlear implant candidacy includes children 1 year or older with bilateral severe to profound sensorineural hearing loss or those aged between 9 and 12 months with bilateral profound sensorineural hearing loss who fail to improve with hearing aid trials. With increasing evidence of early implantation benefit and favorable safety profile in infants, cochlear implantation age was first changed from 24 months to 12 months in 2000 and most recently further lowered to 9 months in May 2020. A study of 403 children with congenital bilateral severe to profound hearing loss examined the effect of age at implant on speech perception, language, and speech production outcomes.[44] Children implanted younger than 12 months had significantly higher open-set speech perception scores, language standard scores, and speech production outcomes. These children also demonstrated language performance within the normative range by school entry with 81% attending mainstream schools.[43]

In addition to children with bilateral sensorineural hearing loss, since 2019, FDA has expanded the indications of cochlear implantation to children 5 years or old with (1) single-sided deafness (SSD) who have profound sensorineural hearing loss in one ear and normal hearing or mild sensorineural hearing loss in the other ear or (2) with asymmetric hearing loss who have profound sensorineural hearing loss in one ear and mild to moderately severe sensorineural hearing loss in the other ear, with a difference of at least 15 dB in pure tone averages between ears. Such changes highlight the fact that children with significant unilateral hearing loss indeed face not only difficulties with language and understanding speech in noise but also educational, social, cognitive, and behavioral challenges potentially resulting in poorer quality of life than their peers with normal bilateral hearing. A recent systematic review and meta-analysis evaluated 119 children with SSD showing clinically meaningful improvement in speech perception in noise, sound localization, and patient-reported quality of sound after cochlear implantation. The meta-analysis also found that the duration of deafness among device nonusers was statistically significantly longer than the duration of deafness among regular device users.[45] There are active ongoing researchers in this area to further enhance the cochlear implantation candidate selection.

Bone Conduction Hearing Devices

Another hearing aid option for children with SSD is bone conduction hearing device. Unlike the traditional hearing aid, a bone conduction hearing device bypasses the outer and middle ears and delivers sound directly to the cochlea via vibrations on the temporal bone. Earlier generations of bone conduction hearing devices deliver vibrations from the sound processor to the temporal bone via either direct contact or magnetic connection with the surgical implant. The former design suffers from not uncommon skin infection around the abutment of the implant, whereas the latter design, avoiding the infection concerns, provides attenuated vibration transfer through the intact skin to the subcutaneous implant. A new generation of bone conduction hearing devices separates the external sound processor from the vibration actuator, which becomes part of the surgical implant underneath the skin. This new design addresses both abovementioned shortcomings of the earlier generations of bone conduction hearing aids. In case of SSD, the sound wave in the form of bone vibration is perceived by the functioning cochlea of the contralateral ear. In other words, one needs to realize that the goal of the fitting bone conduction hearing device in children with SSD is to provide sound awareness, as opposed to sound localization and improved sound discrimination in noise, which can be achieved with cochlear implantation.

Auditory Brainstem Implants

The auditory brainstem implant (ABI) was first developed in 1979 by the House Ear Institute and provides auditory rehabilitation to patients with deafness who are ineligible for cochlear implant surgery due to abnormalities of the cochlea and cochlear nerve. The modern ABI is a multichannel surface array that electrically stimulates second-order neurons in the cochlear nucleus (CN). Compared with the highly tonotopic spiral ganglion in the cochlea, the delineation of neural pathway in CN remains unpredictable and less accurate.[46] Therefore, it is not surprising that the current generation of ABIs provides highly variable and often unpredictable audiometric outcomes. In the United States, there are 3 active FDA trials (Boston, New York, and Los Angeles) evaluating the clinical safety and efficacy of ABI in pediatric patients who have deafness due to severe cochlear anomalies, have cochlear nerve disorders, and do not have NF2. According to an update of the clinical trial in Boston, both primary and revision ABI surgery in children were performed successfully without any major or minor complications. All children achieved environmental sound awareness, and several demonstrated babbling and mimicry.[47] With the estimated study completion date around May 2022, more clinical data will potentially allow the ABI candidacy for children to come down to 18 months of age.

Aural Rehabilitation

Language outcomes will depend on the type of hearing loss, age at which hearing loss occurred, residual hearing, and age at which deficit detection and treatment is initiated. Early intervention program services are available to aid children with hearing loss to learn language and other important cognitive skills. According to the CDC, infants diagnosed with hearing loss should begin their intervention no later than age 6 months, for there are certain critical periods for language development.[48] The American Speech-Language-Hearing Association recommends that by age 3 years, an Individualized Education Program should be implemented, which incorporates audiology services and speech-language pathology services. Services are available through the Individuals with Disabilities Education Improvement Act of 2004, which includes special education programs for school-aged children within the public school system.[49]

The goals of aural rehabilitation are (1) training auditory perception, (2) improving speech, (3) developing language, (4) managing communication, and (5) managing hearing aids and other devices. Specific services are individualized to the patient's needs and are also influenced by the mode of communication the child is using (auditory-oral, American Sign Language, total communication, cued speech, manually coded English, and so forth). The treatment plan will depend on the age of the child, the age at which hearing was lost, degree of hearing loss, type of hearing loss, and the influence of audiologic devices. During training, audiologists and speech therapists will use a variety of techniques to promote the development of auditory perception, including sound discrimination training and using visual cues to give meaning to different messages such as facial expressions, body language, and the context of the communication. The other area of focus is the motor production of speech including voice quality, speaking rate, breath control, loudness, and speech rhythms.[49] In a recent review, Torppa and Huotilainen[50] found correlations between musical skills and speech and language outcomes in hearing-impaired children and encourage speech therapists to use music therapy in their practices. Despite the fact that this finding lacks large-scale randomized controlled trials, this is an area that can be further researched in efforts to improve speech and language therapy for hearing-impaired children.[50] According to the American Academy of Pediatrics successful early intervention programs for children with hearing loss are family centered, monitor development at 6-month intervals with standardized instruments, provide services both in the home as well as in a medical setting, are sensitive to cultural and language differences, and provide accommodations as needed, conduct regular surveys regarding parent satisfaction, and so on. Therefore, these factors should be important considerations when creating a treatment plan for language development in hearing-impaired children.[5]

SUMMARY

Congenital sensorineural hearing loss is highly prevalent in our population, with a wide variety of causes. The key to clinical management is early detection and intervention, to ensure patients are provided with proper resources to promote language and cognitive development. With expanding genetic knowledge about congenital sensorineural hearing loss, the indiscriminate approach in workup such as nontargeted laboratory screening tests or imaging studies is no longer recommended. Comprehensive genetic evaluation and CMV testing are key components to identify the underlying cause of the hearing loss. Therefore, if there is an implication or suspicion of congenital sensorineural hearing loss, evaluations should include a detailed patient history and examination, comprehensive audiologic evaluation, a genetic consultation, as well as appropriate diagnostic imaging. Treatment and prognosis will depend on age of hearing loss and detection. Management plans will typically include audiology consultation, speech therapy, and hearing aids or other technological devices when applicable. Current clinical and outcome research has provided evidence to broaden indications and eligibility for hearing amplification technologies.

CLINICS CARE POINTS

- Being the most common sensory deficit, congenital hearing loss has a prevalence of 1.2 to 1.7 individuals per 1000 live births in the United States. About 20% to 30% of those affected children have profound hearing loss.

- Ongoing advancement in genetic knowledge allows us to have a better understanding of the increased genetic contribution to congenital sensorineural hearing loss.

- The heterogeneous nature of hereditary hearing loss makes the elucidation of the underlying causes challenging. Hence, a comprehensive genetic evaluation by the geneticist is the cornerstone of clinical workup strategy.

- The importance of early diagnosis and medical intervention to improve developmental outcomes is highlighted by the 1-3-6 guidelines proposed by the American Academy of Pediatrics' Joint Committee on Infant Hearing.

- Ongoing clinical and outcome research has broadened indications and eligibility for hearing amplification technologies such as bone conduction hearing device, cochlear implant, and ABI.

REFERENCES

1. Korver AM, Smith RJ, Van Camp G, et al. Congenital hearing loss. Nat Rev Dis Primers 2017;3:16094.
2. Paludetti G, Conti G, DIN W, et al. Infant hearing loss: from diagnosis to therapy Official Report of XXI Conference of Italian Society of Pediatric Otorhinolaryngology. Acta Otorhinolaryngol Ital 2012;32(6):347–70.
3. Ahmadmehrabi S, Li B, Epstein DJ, et al. How does the "cookie-bite" audiogram shape perform in discriminating genetic hearing loss in adults? Otolaryngol Head Neck Surg 2021. https://doi.org/10.1177/01945998211015181. 1945998211015181.
4. Yoshinaga-Itano C, Sedey AL, Coulter DK, et al. Language of early- and later-identified children with hearing loss. Pediatrics 1998;102(5):1161–71.
5. American Academy of Pediatrics JCoIH. Year 2007 position statement: Principles and guidelines for early hearing detection and intervention programs. Pediatrics 2007;120(4):898–921.
6. Lieu JEC, Kenna M, Anne S, et al. Hearing loss in children: a review. JAMA 2020; 324(21):2195–205.
7. Shearer AE, Hildebrand MS, Smith RJH. Hereditary Hearing Loss and Deafness Overview. In: Adam MP, Ardinger HH, Pagon RA, et al., eds GeneReviews((R)). University of Washington, Seattle (WA); 2017.
8. Ko H, Dehority W, Maxwell J R. The impact of maternal infection on the neonate. IntechOpen; 2021.
9. Smith RJ, Bale JF Jr, White KR. Sensorineural hearing loss in children. Lancet 2005;365(9462):879–90.
10. Toriello HV, Smith SD. Hereditary hearing loss and its syndromes. 3rd edition. Oxford University Press; 2016.
11. Marazita ML, Ploughman LM, Rawlings B, et al. Genetic epidemiological studies of early-onset deafness in the U.S. school-age population. Am J Med Genet 1993; 46(5):486–91.
12. Pandya A, Arnos KS, Xia XJ, et al. Frequency and distribution of GJB2 (connexin 26) and GJB6 (connexin 30) mutations in a large North American repository of deaf probands. Genet Med 2003;5(4):295–303.
13. Zhao HB, Kikuchi T, Ngezahayo A, et al. Gap junctions and cochlear homeostasis. J Membr Biol 2006;209(2–3):177–86.
14. Saez JC, Berthoud VM, Branes MC, et al. Plasma membrane channels formed by connexins: their regulation and functions. Physiol Rev 2003;83(4):1359–400.
15. Chan DK, Schrijver I, Chang KW. Connexin-26-associated deafness: phenotypic variability and progression of hearing loss. Genet Med 2010;12(3):174–81.
16. Kenna MA, Feldman HA, Neault MW, et al. Audiologic phenotype and progression in GJB2 (Connexin 26) hearing loss. Arch Otolaryngol Head Neck Surg 2010;136(1):81–7.
17. Norris VW, Arnos KS, Hanks WD, et al. Does universal newborn hearing screening identify all children with GJB2 (Connexin 26) deafness? Penetrance of GJB2 deafness. Ear Hear 2006;27(6):732–41.
18. Snoeckx RL, Huygen PL, Feldmann D, et al. GJB2 mutations and degree of hearing loss: a multicenter study. Am J Hum Genet 2005;77(6):945–57.
19. Sindura KP, Banerjee M. An Immunological Perspective to Non-syndromic Sensorineural Hearing Loss. Front Immunol 2019;10:2848.
20. Moore JK, Linthicum FH Jr. The human auditory system: a timeline of development. Int J Audiol 2007;46(9):460–78.

21. Boppana SB, Ross SA, Fowler KB. Congenital cytomegalovirus infection: clinical outcome. Clin Infect Dis 2013;57(Suppl 4):S178–81.
22. Reef SE, Redd SB, Abernathy E, et al. Evidence used to support the achievement and maintenance of elimination of rubella and congenital rubella syndrome in the United States. J Infect Dis 2011;204(Suppl 2):S593–7.
23. Plotkin SA. The history of rubella and rubella vaccination leading to elimination. Clin Infect Dis 2006;43(Suppl 3):S164–8.
24. Prevention CfDCa. Congenital CMV Infection. 2020. Available at: https://www.cdc.gov/cmv/clinical/congenital-cmv.html.
25. Pass RF, Anderson B. Mother-to-Child Transmission of Cytomegalovirus and Prevention of Congenital Infection. J Pediatr Infect Dis Soc 2014;3(Suppl 1):S2–6.
26. Dollard SC, Grosse SD, Ross DS. New estimates of the prevalence of neurological and sensory sequelae and mortality associated with congenital cytomegalovirus infection. Rev Med Virol 2007;17(5):355–63.
27. Yamamoto AY, Mussi-Pinhata MM, Isaac Mde L, et al. Congenital cytomegalovirus infection as a cause of sensorineural hearing loss in a highly immune population. Pediatr Infect Dis J 2011;30(12):1043–6.
28. Morton CC, Nance WE. Newborn hearing screening–a silent revolution. N Engl J Med 2006;354(20):2151–64.
29. Goderis J, De Leenheer E, Smets K, et al. Hearing loss and congenital CMV infection: a systematic review. Pediatrics 2014;134(5):972–82.
30. Fowler KB, Dahle AJ, Boppana SB, et al. Newborn hearing screening: will children with hearing loss caused by congenital cytomegalovirus infection be missed? J Pediatr 1999;135(1):60–4.
31. Preciado DA, Lawson L, Madden C, et al. Improved diagnostic effectiveness with a sequential diagnostic paradigm in idiopathic pediatric sensorineural hearing loss. Otol Neurotol 2005;26(4):610–5.
32. Belcher R, Virgin F, Duis J, et al. Genetic and Non-genetic Workup for Pediatric Congenital Hearing Loss. Front Pediatr 2021;9:536730.
33. Liming BJ, Carter J, Cheng A, et al. International Pediatric Otolaryngology Group (IPOG) consensus recommendations: Hearing loss in the pediatric patient. Int J Pediatr Otorhinolaryngol 2016;90:251–8.
34. Robin NH. It does matter: the importance of making the diagnosis of a genetic syndrome. Curr Opin Pediatr 2006;18(6):595–7.
35. Estivill X, Govea N, Barcelo E, et al. Familial progressive sensorineural deafness is mainly due to the mtDNA A1555G mutation and is enhanced by treatment of aminoglycosides. Am J Hum Genet 1998;62(1):27–35.
36. Kenneson A, Cannon MJ. Review and meta-analysis of the epidemiology of congenital cytomegalovirus (CMV) infection. Rev Med Virol 2007;17(4):253–76.
37. Adam MP, Ardinger HH, Pagon RA, et al., editors. GeneReviews® [Internet]. Seattle (WA): University of Washington, Seattle; 1993-2022. Available from: https://www.ncbi.nlm.nih.gov/books/NBK1116/
38. Genetic Testing Registry. National Center for Biotechnology Information UNLoM. Available at: https://www.ncbi.nlm.nih.gov/gtr/.
39. Chen YS, Emmerling O, Ilgner J, et al. Idiopathic sudden sensorineural hearing loss in children. Int J Pediatr Otorhinolaryngol 2005;69(6):817–21.
40. Prosser JD, Cohen AP, Greinwald JH. Diagnostic Evaluation of Children with Sensorineural Hearing Loss. Otolaryngol Clin North Am 2015;48(6):975–82.
41. Sininger YS, Grimes A, Christensen E. Auditory development in early amplified children: factors influencing auditory-based communication outcomes in children with hearing loss. Ear Hear 2010;31(2):166–85.

42. Audiology AAo. Clinical Practice Guidelines: Pediatric Amplification. Available at: https://audiology-web.s3.amazonaws.com/migrated/PediatricAmplification Guidelines.pdf_539975b3e7e9f1.74471798.pdf.

43. Disorders NIoDaOC. Cochlear Implants. Published 2016. Available at https://www.nidcd.nih.gov/health/cochlear-implants.

44. Dettman SJ, Dowell RC, Choo D, et al. Long-term Communication Outcomes for Children Receiving Cochlear Implants Younger Than 12 Months: A Multicenter Study. Otol Neurotol 2016;37(2):e82–95.

45. Benchetrit L, Ronner EA, Anne S, et al. Cochlear Implantation in Children With Single-Sided Deafness: A Systematic Review and Meta-analysis. JAMA Otolaryngol Head Neck Surg 2021;147(1):58–69.

46. Wong K, Kozin ED, Kanumuri VV, et al. Auditory Brainstem Implants: Recent Progress and Future Perspectives. Front Neurosci 2019;13:10.

47. Puram SV, Barber SR, Kozin ED, et al. Outcomes following Pediatric Auditory Brainstem Implant Surgery: Early Experiences in a North American Center. Otolaryngol Head Neck Surg 2016;155(1):133–8.

48. Prevention CfDCa. Hearing Loss Treatment and Intervention Services. 2020. Available at: https://www.cdc.gov/ncbddd/hearingloss/treatment.html.

49. The American Speech-Language-Hearing Association. Child Aural/Audiologic Rehabilitation. 2021. Available at: https://www.asha.org/public/hearing/child-aural-rehabilitation/. Accessed October 20, 2021.

50. Torppa R, Huotilainen M. Why and how music can be used to rehabilitate and develop speech and language skills in hearing-impaired children. Hear Res 2019;380:108–22.

Ankyloglossia and Tethered Oral Tissue

An Evidence-Based Review

Guy Talmor, MD[a,1], Christen L. Caloway, MD[a,b],*

KEYWORDS

- Ankyloglossia • Tongue tie • Pediatric otolaryngology

KEY POINTS

- Ankyloglossia may result in feeding and speech impairment.
- Frenotomy is most beneficial in improving maternal comfort during breastfeeding.
- The benefit of intervention for posterior ankyloglossia and labial frenula remains unclear.

INTRODUCTION

While ankyloglossia may present along a spectrum of anatomic variation or true pathologic restriction of the movement of the tongue, it nonetheless is a frequent cause of both feeding and speech difficulties in young children. Ankyloglossia, or tongue-tie, was described as early as 350 BC, when Aristotle opined that in "the case of those whose tongues are slightly tied: their speech is indistinct and lisping."[1,2] Then, in the 1600s, techniques for tongue-tie release were published in textbooks.[3] Early instrumentation for frenulotomy used scissors and, in some cases, fingernails. Midwives were reported to use an intentionally overgrown fingernail when lysing lingual attachments.[4] In the age of modern medicine, procedural intervention for ankyloglossia is performed by physicians across several medical specialties.[5]

The prevalence of ankyloglossia is highly variable in the literature. Some reports place the prevalence at under 1%, while others estimate prevalence to be as high as 10% to 12%.[6–8] This variability reflects the absence of clear diagnostic criteria for ankyloglossia and the subjective, examination-dependent nature of the diagnosis. Despite this inconsistency in the literature, it is rather clear that ankyloglossia has been diagnosed and treated at a higher rate in recent years. In a national database review, Walsh and colleagues[9] found that the diagnosis of ankyloglossia increased nearly 10-fold from 1997 to 2012. Frenotomy rates similarly increased during that time. With

[a] Department of Otolaryngology–Head and Neck Surgery, Rutgers-New Jersey Medical School, 90 Bergen Street, Suite 8100, Newark, NJ 07103, USA; [b] Department of Surgery, St. Joseph's University Medical Center, 11 Getty Avenue, Paterson, NJ 07503, USA
[1] Present address: 230 Bloomfield Street #401, Hoboken, NJ 07030.
* Corresponding author. 11 Getty Avenue, Paterson, NJ 07503.
E-mail address: calowayc@sjhmc.org

Pediatr Clin N Am 69 (2022) 235–245
https://doi.org/10.1016/j.pcl.2021.12.007
0031-3955/22/© 2021 Elsevier Inc. All rights reserved.

pediatric.theclinics.com

increasing intervention rates, it becomes essential for providers to accurately diagnose ankyloglossia and determine which patients would benefit most from frenotomy. The goal of this chapter is to provide an overview of the embryology, diagnosis, and treatment of ankyloglossia as well as other oral ties with particular emphasis on patient selection and candidacy for intervention.

Embryology

Tongue formation begins around the fourth week of gestation. As reflected by its complex innervation patterns, the tongue develops from the first, second, third, and fourth pharyngeal arches. This begins with the tuberculum impar, an outgrowth of the first arch that is subsequently accompanied by symmetric lateral swellings. These eventually overgrow the tuberculum and fuse to form the anterior tongue. Median swellings from the other arches, also referred to as the hypobranchial eminence, grow and eventually comprise the posterior tongue. The developing tongue is made up of several cell types, including myocytes as well as neural crest derivatives that ultimately form connective tissue.[10] As the tongue develops, it separates from the floor of mouth. This process is characterized by cellular degeneration, resulting in the formation of the lingual sulcus. Ankyloglossia results from a failure in the cellular degeneration of the frenulum, which results in a fibrous band anchoring the tongue to the floor of mouth. This band may be present along the anterior surface of the ventral tongue, or may be more intrinsically associated with tongue musculature, which is known as "posterior ankyloglossia."[11] This entity will be further discussed later in the text.

Presentation and Diagnosis

Ankyloglossia represents a challenge to providers given the absence of universal diagnostic criteria. It is most frequently noted when feeding difficulty develops shortly after birth. In many cases, maternal symptomatology is the inciting factor that leads to a thorough oral examination that diagnoses ankyloglossia. A full review of the mechanism of breastfeeding is beyond the scope of this chapter. Briefly, tethering of the anterior tongue is thought to weaken the infant's ability to latch onto the nipple. Furthermore, it may impair the formation of a proper seal. Sonographic studies suggest that breastfeeding is dependent on the formation of a vacuum, resulting in the downstream flow of milk.[12] Tethering of the tongue impairs this vacuum. Clinically, this results in several noticeable changes to the mother, the most prominent of which is mastalgia. This may also lead to cracking, fissuring, and ulceration of the nipple. Feeds are often prolonged as well.

The association of ankyloglossia with other syndromes such as Ehlers-Danlos and Ellis-van Creveld mandates that a full physical examination is performed to rule out other craniofacial abnormalities.[13] Examination should note resting tongue position, and, if possible, elicit protrusion from the patient. This is particularly difficult given the likely constraints due to patient age, and often a comprehensive feeding evaluation is needed for proper functional examination.[14] The lingual frenulum is often best examined using manual retraction. In the author's experience, this is best performed when an assistant controls the infant head position and the examiner can retract the tongue superiorly with both forefingers. A thorough oral examination is then performed to assess for neonatal teeth, cleft palate, and other oral ties such as the presence of a labial frenulum.

It is imperative that the provider diagnosing ankyloglossia recognize that feeding is a complex process that depends on both behavioral and anatomic characteristics of the infant and mother. Ankyloglossia may, indeed, result in feeding difficulty. Functional impairments caused by ankyloglossia may include reduced range of motion, tongue clicking, loss of seal, and/or creased or misshapen nipples after feeding.[14] Other anatomic abnormalities, such as cleft lip and palate, are readily apparent on examination.[15] More subtle abnormalities include neurologic deficits, weak reflexes, detrimental biting patterns, prior placement of an enteric feeding tube and alterations in tongue position.[16] These must be reliably excluded when determining eligibility for interventions such as frenotomy. A comprehensive feeding evaluation may assess for other causes of feeding difficulty, including challenges with sleep state regulation, hunger state regulation, breastfeeding latch, volume or rate of breastmilk flow, physical discomfort due to reflux, and/or parental anxiety surrounding breastfeeding.[14]

In older children, ankyloglossia may present with speech impairment. The true impact of oral ties on speech production remains controversial. Some have postulated that oral ties, and ankyloglossia, in particular, may affect speech production and intelligibility.[17] However, there is a paucity in confirmational evidence. Daggumati and colleagues[18] compared speech production between patients with treated and untreated ankyloglossia, finding no significant difference. Another cross-sectional study examining speech parameters in treated versus untreated ankyloglossia similarly did not find any significant differences. Therefore, whether ankyloglossia results in true speech impediment remains a topic of considerable debate. Nonetheless, providers should perform a thorough examination, including assessment for oral ties, in older children presenting with impaired speech production or intelligibility. It is also imperative to consult with a trained Speech-Language Pathologist for the comprehensive assessment of oral function and speech production.

Grading

There are several metrics used to grade the severity of ankyloglossia. These grading systems can be broadly classified into anatomic and functional scales. Kotlow's classification focuses on the distance between the frenulum and tip of the anterior tongue, which is inversely correlated with severity (**Table 1**). The Corrylos criteria similarly incorporate the frenulum attachment point onto the tongue but also grade the firmness and shape of the lingual attachment (**Box 1**).[19] The Hazelbaker Assessment Tool for Lingual Frenulum Function (HATLFF) is a frequently cited tool designed to screen for ankyloglossia using both appearance and function.[20] Other functional tools may be used as well, including LATCH (Latch, Audible swallowing, nipple Type, Comfort Hold) and Infant Breastfeeding Assessment Tool (IBFAT) to determine breastfeeding competence and identify any difficulties in the feeding process.[21–23]

Posterior Tongue Tie

Posterior tongue tie remains a controversial and poorly defined clinical entity. To some providers, posterior ankyloglossia represents a thick fibrous band that inserts posteriorly into the ventral tongue. Others believe it to represent a submucosal fibrous band

Table 1	
Kotlow criteria for ankyloglossia based on free tongue length anterior to frenulum attachment	
Clinically Normal	**<16 mm**
Class I. Mild Ankyloglossia	12–16 mm
Class II. Moderate Ankyloglossia	8–11 mm
Class III. Severe Ankyloglossia	3–7 mm
Class IV. Complete Ankyloglossia	<3 mm

Box 1
Coryllos ankyloglossia classification

Type 1. Insertion of the frenulum to the tip of the tongue

Type 2. Insertion of the frenulum 2–4 mm posterior to the tip of the tongue

Type 3. Thickened frenulum attached to the mid-tongue and the middle of the floor of mouth, tight and less elastic

Type 4. Thick, shiny inelastic submucosal frenulum that restricts movement at the base of the tongue

---

that is thus obscured from visual inspection and can only be palpated.[24,25] A panel of pediatric otolaryngologists discussed the topic and were unable to achieve a proper consensus on the definition of posterior ankyloglossia. Certain providers even felt that posterior ankyloglossia does not represent a true clinical entity and should be disregarded altogether.[26] Given the ill-defined nature of this diagnosis, robust evidence showing the benefit of frenotomy for posterior ankyloglossia is lacking. Prior studies have shown higher revision rates for patients undergoing frenotomy for posterior ankyloglossia.[27] In a recent randomized trial, Ghaheri and colleagues[11] demonstrated improved breastfeeding efficacy, including rhythmic coordinated movement and tongue speed, in patients undergoing frenotomy for posterior ankyloglossia compared with untreated controls. Studies are limited by sample size and often vary in methodology, necessitating that further research is dedicated to this clinical entity in the future.

Other Oral Ties

Other oral ties have been reported in the literature. The most frequently discussed oral tie following ankyloglossia has been the labial frenulum, or lip tie. Specifically, the upper lip tie extends from the lip to the maxillary gingiva. Like ankyloglossia, Kotlow proposed a grading system for upper lip tie based on attachment position.[28] (**Box 2**) The most severe cases involve the insertion of the labial frenulum between the central incisors. Theoretically, upper lip tie can reduce lip flanging and result in weaker latch.[29] Some have proposed that upper lip ties contribute to the formation of dental caries as they promote stasis and deposition by creating defined pockets along the maxillary incisors.[30] Another oral tie discussed in the literature is the buccal tie. This term refers to tissue thickening between the buccal mucosa and the mandibular or maxillary alveolar ridge. Buccal ties are most frequently noted in the region of the canines or premolars.[23] Evidence regarding the division of buccal ties is lacking in the literature.

Box 2
Kotlow criteria for labial frenula

Type 1. Normal

Type 2. Insertion of the frenulum between or just above the central incisors

Type 3. Frenulum beginning to insert into the anterior papilla

Type 4. Frenulum insertion into anterior papilla

DISCUSSION
Treatment

Intervention for ankyloglossia is primarily performed for feeding difficulty. Later in life, it may be pursued for speech impediment.[31] When addressing feeding difficulty, the primary treatment options are the division of the frenulum or supportive care, which is usually accomplished with feeding support through lactation consultants and myofunctional therapy.[1] Feeding support is accomplished through alterations in positioning and devices such as nipple shields. In older patients, myofunctional therapy may be helpful in correcting maladaptive oral patterns while promoting awareness of oral and tongue posture. Myofunctional therapy has been applied in an adjunctive postfrenotomy manner as well. In most patients, especially those with feeding difficulty, the treatment option of choice is the division of the frenulum.[32]

Candidates for Operative Intervention

Surgical options for ankyloglossia include frenotomy and, in more involved cases, frenuloplasty and frenectomy.[33] These procedures are regarded as relatively straightforward from a technical aspect with a favorable safety profile.[1] The challenge is determining the appropriate candidate for these procedures. A continuation of the prevalence study by Walsh, Xie and colleagues[34] demonstrated that the diagnosis of ankyloglossia and the number of procedures that were subsequently performed has continued to increase greatly in recent years. This trend has led to speculation ankyloglossia is over-treated and that, in some instances, frenotomy may be offered in cases whereby conservative management and feeding support would otherwise be sufficient. In this section, we will review the evidence regarding surgical intervention for ankyloglossia in an effort to better elucidate the cases in which intervention is indicated and beneficial for the mother-infant dyad.

Studies examining the efficacy of intervention for ankyloglossia are highly variable in grading, methodology, and outcome measurements. Hogan and colleagues[35] randomized patients to frenotomy or supportive care, with significant improvement in feeding following frenotomy. Dollberg and colleagues[20] attempted to compare patients undergoing frenotomy versus sham procedures and did not find significant improvement in LATCH scores. Nonetheless, maternal nipple pain was significantly improved following frenotomy. A similarly constructed study found improved breastfeeding and maternal pain following frenotomy. Interestingly, maternal pain scores in this study improved following sham surgery, indicating the possibility of a placebo effect component in these results[36] Similarly, Berry reported immediate improvement in maternal pain and perceived feeding, although an objective observer did not note significant improvement in feeding on examination when comparing patients with frenotomy to control groups.[37] In a larger randomized controlled trial, Emond and colleagues[38] found that HATLFF scores improved following frenotomy, but functional scores such as LATCH and IBFAT did not find significantly differ from controls. As previously mentioned, there is great variability in the methodology used in these studies. This variability partially stems from the lack of a consensus definition for ankyloglossia. While some studies relied on objective screening tools such as the HATLFF, other studies recruited patients based on their own definitions of ankyloglossia, often relating to physical examination findings such as tongue protrusion or site of frenulum insertion relative to the anterior tip of the tongue. Furthermore, many of these studies had different outcome measurements, with some using objective examination of feeding efficacy while others used standardized tools such as the IBFAT and LATCH. As such, it is difficult to draw wide-ranging conclusions from the current literature on frenotomy. Perhaps the most consistent finding in the literature is a decrease in maternal pain with feeding, which, as supported by Buryk and colleagues,[34] may partially arise from the placebo effect. Systematic reviews have echoed these conclusions and were only able to reliably mention alleviation of maternal pain during breastfeeding, noting that heterogeneity in methodology and the relatively small number of randomized controlled trials precluded the authors from drawing more wide-ranging conclusions on the benefits of frenotomy.[39,40] As mentioned previously, given the lack of evidence confirming the detrimental impact of ankyloglossia on speech production, there are currently no clear guidelines indicating which patients would benefit from frenotomy to address speech impairment.

Surgical Intervention

Once patients are deemed eligible candidates, the surgeon has several options at their disposal to address a lingual frenulum. These options vary in both technique and instrumentation. Cold steel division of the tissue has the lowest risk to the surrounding tissues; however, hemostasis is often a challenge. The use of silver nitrate or electrocautery for hemostasis reintroduces a risk of burn to surrounding tissue. Monopolar electrocautery is effective but has a risk of burn injury to surrounding tissues. Furthermore, grounding in the patient is often necessary. Bipolar electrocautery is more directed; however, the risk of burn injury is still present. Laser has the key advantages of limited bleeding and reduced scarring, but this technique is both expensive and requires an experienced team and standardized precautions to ensure safe use and minimize fire risk.

The most widely used and simple intervention for ankyloglossia is frenotomy. This procedure is the simple release of the frenulum with no subsequent tissue arrangement.[32] Contraindications include bleeding disorders and failure to receive Vitamin K at birth for infants. In more involved procedures, patients deemed at high risk for general anesthesia may not be ideal candidates.[41] The frenulum is divided without the need to breach muscle tissue. Frenotomy is frequently performed at the bedside or clinical setting without the need for general anesthesia. Division may be performed with sharp instrumentation such as a blade or scissors as well as electrocautery and laser. No randomized controlled trials comparing cold steel, electrocautery, and laser frenotomy have been published in the literature. Given that tissues are lysed without tissue rearrangement, frenotomy theoretically has a risk of scarring and reformation of the lingual frenulum. Therefore, more advanced techniques were designed to mitigate this risk.

Frenuloplasty is a more extensive procedure reserved for severe ankyloglossia or revision cases. This procedure is more involved and typically requires the use of general anesthesia. The simplest form of frenuloplasty involves a similar incision to the basic frenotomy that is subsequently carried posteriorly into the muscular tissue of the tongue, resulting in a vertically-oriented defect that is closed primarily.[42] More extensive techniques can be used, including a two-flap Z-plasty. This technique requires the surgeon to make the aforementioned incision along the frenulum and then create 2 equal opposing incisions that extend from the resulting midline vertical defect at a 45 to 60° angle, forming a "Z." Once these incisions are made, 2 separate flaps can be elevated, rotated and sutured in place. A four-flap variation of this procedure exists as well and is preferred by some providers.[43] These procedures are thought to potentially reduce the risk of scarring and revision at the expense of a more involved procedure that requires general anesthesia. With more soft tissue dissection and anatomic disruption, there may be more potential for postoperative pain and bleeding.

The literature comparing ankyloglossia release techniques is scarce. Kim and colleagues compared frenotomy and four-flap frenuloplasty in children with speech articulation difficulty. No significant differences in speech production were found between the 2 interventions.[44] In a systematic review of ankyloglossia release techniques, Khan and colleagues[45] did not find any clear evidence demonstrating the benefit of Z-plasty over other frenuloplasty or frenotomy techniques.

Treatment of Posterior Tongue Tie

Reflective of the ambiguity surrounding posterior tongue tie and debate regarding its true definition, the evidence supporting posterior tongue tie release is sparse. In a noncontrolled study, Ghaheri and colleagues[46] demonstrated improved breastfeeding outcomes, including total intake, once frenotomy was performed for both anterior and posterior ankyloglossia. A subsequent randomized controlled trial by the same author exclusively evaluating patients with posterior ankyloglossia similarly found improvement in objective feeding metrics as well as reduced maternal pain following frenotomy.[11] The initial diagnosis was based on targeted clinical examination as no well-defined screening tools have been proposed for posterior ankyloglossia. Until a clinical consensus is reached on the diagnosis of posterior ankyloglossia, the need for intervention will have to be determined at the provider's discretion on a case-by-case basis.

Treatment of Other Oral Ties

The body of evidence supporting the division of other oral ties is even further limited by sample size and variability in methodology. Following the lingual frenulum, most attention in the literature is directed toward the labial frenulum, or upper lip tie. There are few studies that exclusively examine the effect of labial frenotomy on speech and swallow outcomes. Most studies investigating the release of a lip tie often do so in conjunction with release of tongue tie, thus obscuring whether any possible patient benefits occurred due to the release of the tongue tie, lip tie, or both. Pransky and colleagues reported improvement in breastfeeding following lip tie release, but many patients also underwent tongue tie release, leading the authors to concede that a clear link between lip tie and feeding difficulty could not be drawn due to its copresentation and simultaneous treatment with other oral ties.[47] In a nonrandomized pilot study by Patel and colleagues,[48] mothers reported subjective improvements in breastfeeding following isolated lip tie release. However, this study was limited by small sample size and lack of control group. Attempting to address the limitations in small, single-institution studies, Nakhash and colleagues conducted a systemic review of the literature pertaining to upper lip tie. They did not find any clear evidence for labial frenulum release and were unable to demonstrate any benefit with regards to breastfeeding outcomes.[49] The limited evidence behind lip tie treatment has led providers to issue statements cautioning others against the aggressive treatment of lip ties.[50] Given the limited evidence demonstrating the benefit of labial frenotomy, providers are cautioned to selectively determine which patients would benefit most from this procedure.

SUMMARY

Ankyloglossia can lead to impediments in breastfeeding and eventually speech articulation. Despite the prevalence of ankyloglossia and increased incidence in recent years, there remains paucity in the literature confirming the wide-ranging benefits of frenotomy. Perhaps the clearest benefit of frenotomy is improvement in maternal comfort during breastfeeding. Further randomized controlled trials are necessary to determine whether frenotomy offers clear benefits in terms of infant breastfeeding metrics and overall efficiency and intake. There are a variety of tools and techniques available for the treatment of ankyloglossia, with no clear evidence confirming the superiority of one technique over the others. The definition of other oral ties such as posterior ankyloglossia and the labial frenulum remains debated in the literature. Evidence regarding the surgical treatment of these entities is limited, and providers should exercise caution to avoid overtreatment of these oral ties.

CLINICS CARE POINTS

- The prevalence of ankyloglossia and utilization of frenotomy has increased in recent years.
- The clearest benefit of frenotomy is improvement in maternal comfort during breastfeeding.
- There is equivocal evidence regarding improvements in breastfeeding and speech metrics following frenotomy.
- Studies investigating frenotomy are variable in methodology, thus making it difficult to draw wide-ranging conclusions regarding the benefits of this procedure.
- Systematic reviews have found low to insufficient evidence for meaningful conclusions regarding the benefit of intervention for ankyloglossia.
- There is no clear evidence demonstrating improved feeding and speech articulation following frenulectomy or frenuloplasty versus conventional frenotomy.
- Posterior ankyloglossia is a poorly defined clinical entity and evidence supporting its treatment is poor.
- Labial frenulum, or upper lip tie, has been suspected to impair breastfeeding and increase the risk of dental caries, although clear evidence supporting labial frenotomy is scarce.

DISCLOSURES

The authors have nothing to disclose.

REFERENCES

1. Walsh J, McKenna Benoit M. Ankyloglossia and other oral ties. Otolaryngol Clin North Am 2019;52(5):795–811.
2. Patel J, Anthonappa RP, King NM. All tied up! Influences of oral frenulae on breastfeeding and their recommended management strategies. J Clin Pediatr Dent 2018;42(6):407–13.
3. Scultetus, J. Wund-artzneyisches Zeug-Hauss 1679.
4. Horton CE, Crawford HH, Adamson JE, et al. Tongue-tie. Cleft Palate J 1969; 6:8–23.
5. Solis-Pazmino P, Kim GS, Lincango-Naranjo E, et al. Major complications after tongue-tie release: A case report and systematic review. Int J Pediatr Otorhinolaryngol 2020;138:110356.
6. Becker S, Mendez MD. Ankyloglossia. 2021. In: StatPearls [Internet]. Treasure Island, FL: StatPearls Publishing; 2021.
7. Ankur K, Joshi C, Prasad A, et al. Prevalence of tongue-tie in infants weighing≥1800gat birth. Indian J Pediatr 2021;88(10):1057.
8. Rech RS, Chávez BA, Fernandez PB, et al. Presence of ankyloglossia and breastfeeding in babies born in Lima, Peru: a longitudinal study. Codas 2021;32(6): e20190235.

9. Walsh J, Links A, Boss E, et al. Ankyloglossia and lingual frenotomy: National Trends in inpatient diagnosis and management in the United States, 1997-2012. Otolaryngol Head Neck Surg 2017;156(4):735–40.

10. Parada C, Han, Chai Y. Molecular and cellular regulatory mechanisms of tongue myogenesis. J Dent Res 2012;91(6):528–35. https://doi.org/10.1177/0022034511434055.

11. Ghaheri BA, Lincoln D, Mai TNT, et al. Objective improvement after frenotomy for posterior tongue-tie: a prospective randomized trial. Otolaryngol Head Neck Surg 2021. 1945998211039784.

12. Geddes DT, Kent JC, Mitoulas LR, et al. Tongue movement and intra-oral vacuum in breastfeeding infants. Early Hum Dev 2008;84(7):471–7.

13. Mintz SM, Siegel MA, Seider PJ. An overview of oral frena and their association with multiple syndromic and nonsyndromic conditions. Oral Surg Oral Med Oral Pathol Oral Radiol Endod 2005;99(3):321–4.

14. Caloway C, Hersh CJ, Baars R, et al. Association of feeding evaluation with frenotomy rates in infants with breastfeeding difficulties. JAMA Otolaryngol Head Neck Surg 2019;145(9):817–22.

15. Sanches MT. Manejo clínico das disfunções orais na amamentação [Clinical management of oral disorders in breastfeeding]. J Pediatr Suppl 2004;80(5):S155–62.

16. Flint A, New K, Davies MW. Cup feeding versus other forms of supplemental enteral feeding for newborn infants unable to fully breastfeed. Cochrane Database Syst Rev 2016;2016(8):CD005092.

17. Shen T, Sie KC. Surgical speech disorders. Facial Plast Surg Clin North Am 2014;22(4):593–609.

18. Daggumati S, Cohn JE, Brennan MJ, et al. Caregiver perception of speech quality in patients with ankyloglossia: comparison between surgery and non-treatment. Int J Pediatr Otorhinolaryngol 2019;119:70–4.

19. Genna CW, Coryllos EV. Breastfeeding and tongue-tie. J Hum Lact 2009;25(1):111–2.

20. Hazelbaker AK. Newborn tongue-tie and breast-feeding. J Am Board Fam 2005;18(4):326–7.

21. Riordan J, Bibb D, Miller M, et al. Predicting breastfeeding duration using the LATCH breastfeeding assessment tool. J Hum Lact 2001;17(1):20–3.

22. Riordan JM, Koehn M. Reliability and validity testing of three breastfeeding assessment tools. J Obstet Gynecol Neonatal Nurs 1997;26(2):181–7.

23. Dollberg S, Botzer E, Grunis E, et al. Immediate nipple pain relief after frenotomy in breast-fed infants with ankyloglossia: a randomized, prospective study. J Pediatr Surg 2006;41(9):1598–600.

24. Mills N, Keough N, Geddes DT, et al. Defining the anatomy of the neonatal lingual frenulum. Clin Anat 2019;32(6):824–35.

25. Ruffoli R, Giambelluca MA, Scavuzzo MC, et al. Ankyloglossia: a morphofunctional investigation in children. Oral Dis 2005;11(3):170–4.

26. Messner AH, Walsh J, Rosenfeld RM, et al. Clinical consensus statement: ankyloglossia in children. Otolaryngol Head Neck Surg 2020;162(5):597–611.

27. Hong P, Lago D, Seargeant J, et al. Defining ankyloglossia: a case series of anterior and posterior tongue ties. Int J Pediatr Otorhinolaryngol 2010;74(9):1003–6.

28. Kotlow LA. Diagnosing and understanding the maxillary lip-tie (superior labial, the maxillary labial frenum) as it relates to breastfeeding. J Hum Lact 2013;29(4):458–64.

29. Kotlow L. Infant reflux and aerophagia associated with the maxillary lip-tie and ankyloglossia (tongue-tie). Clin Lact 2011;2(4):25–9.

30. Kotlow LA. The influence of the maxillary frenum on the development and pattern of dental caries on anterior teeth in breastfeeding infants: preven-tion, diagnosis, and treatment. J Hum Lact 2010;26(3):304–8.

31. Wang J, Yang X, Hao S, et al. The effect of ankyloglossia and tongue-tie division on speech articulation: a systematic review. Int J Paediatr Dent 2021.

32. Zaghi S, Valcu-Pinkerton S, Jabara M, et al. Aug, Lingual frenuloplasty with my-ofunctional therapy: exploring safety and efficacy in 348 cases. Laryngoscope Investig Otolaryngol 2019;4(5):489–96.

33. Lalakea ML, Messner AH. Ankyloglossia: does it matter? Pediatr Clin North Am 2003;50(2):381–97.

34. Wei EX, Tunkel D, Boss E, et al. Ankyloglossia: update on trends in diagnosis and management in the United States, 2012-2016. Otolaryngol Head Neck Surg 2020;163(5):1029–31.

35. Hogan M, Westcott C, Griffiths M. Randomized, controlled trial of division of tongue-tie in infants with feeding problems. J Paediatr Child Health 2005; 41(5–6):246–50.

36. Buryk M, Bloom D, Shope T. Efficacy of neonatal release of ankyloglossia: a ran-domized trial. Pediatrics 2011;128(2):280–8.

37. Berry J, Griffiths M, Westcott C. A double-blind, randomized, controlled trial of tongue-tie division and its immediate effect on breastfeeding. Breastfeed Med 2012;7(3):189–93.

38. Emond A, Ingram J, Johnson D, et al. Randomised controlled trial of early frenot-omy in breastfed infants with mild-moderate tongue-tie. Arch Dis Child Fetal Neonatal Ed 2014;99(3):F189–95.

39. O'Shea JE, Foster JP, O'Donnell CP, et al. Frenotomy for tongue-tie in newborn infants. Cochrane Database Syst Rev 2017;3(3):CD011065.

40. Francis DO, Krishnaswami S, McPheeters M. Treatment of ankyloglossia and breastfeeding outcomes: a systematic review. Pediatrics 2015;135(6): e1458–66.

41. Kenny-Scherber AC, Newman J. Office-based frenotomy for ankyloglossia and problematic breastfeeding. Can Fam Physician 2016;62(7):570–1.

42. Junqueira MA, Cunha NN, Costa e Silva LL, et al. Surgical techniques for the treatment of ankyloglossia in children: a case series. J Appl Oral Sci 2014; 22(3):241–8.

43. Baker AR, Carr MM. Surgical treatment of ankyloglossia. Oper Tech Otolaryngol Head Neck Surg 2015;26(1):28–32.

44. Kim TH, Lee YC, Yoo SD, et al. Comparison of simple frenotomy with 4-flap Z-fre-nuloplasty in treatment for ankyloglossia with articulation difficulty: a prospective randomized study. Int J Pediatr Otorhinolaryngol 2020;136:110146.

45. Khan U, MacPherson J, Bezuhly M, et al. Comparison of frenotomy techniques for the treatment of ankyloglossia in children: a systematic review. Otolaryngol Head Neck Surg 2020;163(3):428–43.

46. Ghaheri BA, Cole M, Fausel SC, et al. Breastfeeding improvement following tongue-tie and lip-tie release: a prospective cohort study. Laryngoscope 2017; 127(5):1217–23.

47. Pransky SM, Lago D, Hong P. Breastfeeding difficulties and oral cavity anomalies: the influence of posterior ankyloglossia and upper-lip ties. Int J Pediatr Otorhino-laryngol 2015;79(10):1714–7.

48. Patel PS, Wu DB, Schwartz Z, et al. Upper lip frenotomy for neonatal breastfeeding problems. Int J Pediatr Otorhinolaryngol 2019;124:190–2.
49. Nakhash R, Wasserteil N, Mimouni FB, et al. Upper lip tie and breastfeeding: a systematic review. Breastfeed Med 2019;14(2):83–7.
50. Fraser L, Benzie S, Montgomery J. Posterior tongue tie and lip tie: a lucrative private industry where the evidence is uncertain. BMJ 2020;371:m3928.

Tonsillectomy and Adenoidectomy - Pediatric Clinics of North America

Brandon K. Nguyen, MD[a], Huma A. Quraishi, MD[b],*

KEYWORDS

- Tonsils • Adenoids • Tonsillitis • Tonsillectomy • Adenoidectomy
- Adenotonsillectomy • Intracapsular tonsillectomy

KEY POINTS

- OSA is the most common indication for adenotonsillectomy.
- PSG is the gold standard for diagnosing OSA.
- Adenotonsillectomy for OSA results in an improvement in obstructive symptoms, behavior, and PSG and QOL measures.
- The Paradise criteria should be used in recommending tonsillectomy for recurrent pharyngitis.
- The indications for adenoidectomy include OSA, chronic otitis media with effusion, and recurrent sinusitis.

INTRODUCTION

Tonsillectomy and adenoidectomy are among the most commonly performed major pediatric operations in the United States, with more than 500,000 procedures performed annually.[1]

This procedure can be performed with or without adenoidectomy. These procedures were traditionally performed for recurrent tonsillitis; however, the vast majority of tonsillectomies are currently performed for obstructive symptoms.[2,3] When performed for appropriate indications, tonsillectomy and adenoidectomy can greatly improve a child's quality of life (QOL) and general health.[4,5] Given the prevalence of these conditions and subsequent surgical procedures, evidence-based recommendations are regularly evaluated and updated.[6] As such, familiarity with these guidelines is

The authors have nothing to disclose and have no financial or commercial conflicts of interest in relation to the preparation of this article.
[a] Department of Otolaryngology–Head and Neck Surgery, Rutgers New Jersey Medical School, 90 Bergen St, Ste 8100, Newark, NJ 07103, USA; [b] Pediatric Otolaryngology, Joseph M. Sanzari Children's Hospital, 30 Prospect Ave. WFAN Bldg 3rd Floor, Hackensack, NJ 07601, USA
* Corresponding author.
E-mail address: huma.quraishi@hmhn.org

necessary for pediatric practitioners. This review summarizes the indications, complications, and outcomes for tonsillectomy and adenoidectomy, as well as provides a brief overview of operative techniques.

Anatomy and Physiology

Tonsils and adenoids play an important role in the host defense against invading inhaled or ingested pathogens. These lymphoid structures are arranged in a circular orientation around the naso- and oropharynx called Waldeyer's ring. This ring consists of the nasopharyngeal tonsil known as the adenoids, the tubal tonsils adjacent to the eustachian tube, the palatine tonsils in the oropharynx, and the lingual tonsils at the base of the tongue.

Tonsils are secondary lymphoepithelial organs that initiate the immune response from antigens entering through the nose or the mouth. These tissues are derivatives of the 2nd pharyngeal pouch, typically arise between the 4th and 5th months of gestation, and continue to develop through birth and childhood.[7,8] The greatest immunologic activity for tonsils typically occurs between 3 and 10 years of age and explains the high incidence of obstructive sleep-disordered breathing and recurrent tonsillitis during these ages.[9]

The adenoid pad is situated in the nasopharynx with the apex just inferior to the nasal septum and the base along the posterior nasopharyngeal wall. The adenoid pad develops as a midline structure by the fusion of 2 lateral primordia in the seventh month of gestation and continues to mature until the fifth or sixth year of life and typically involutes by adolescence.[10,11]

The most widely accepted grading scale for tonsil size was proposed by Brodsky in 1989 (**Table 1**). Multiple trials have confirmed the reproducibility of the Brodsky grading scale. Interestingly, much has been made of tonsil size, but multiple studies have shown that size does not correlate with the degree of obstruction clinically.[12,13]

INDICATIONS FOR TONSILLECTOMY
Obstructive Sleep Apnea Syndrome

Obstructive sleep disorder breathing (oSDB) is one of the primary indications for adenotonsillectomy. oSDB is characterized by either abnormality of the respiratory pattern or adequacy of ventilation during sleep. oSDB encompasses a spectrum of obstructive disorders that range from snoring to obstructive sleep apnea (OSA).[14,15] OSAS is characterized by recurrent partial or complete obstruction of the airway during sleep. Even though the prevalence of snoring is high in the pediatric population, estimated to be 8% to 27%, only 1% to 5% of children will have OSAS.[15] Untreated, pediatric OSA can lead to a myriad of morbidities including daytime sleepiness,

Table 1	
Brodsky tonsil size classification	
Grade	**Ratio of Tonsil in Oropharynx**
0	Tonsils are entirely within the tonsillar pillar or previously resected
1+	Tonsils occupy <25% of the lateral dimension of the oropharynx, as measured between the anterior tonsillar pillars
2+	Tonsils occupy 26%–50% of the lateral dimension of the oropharynx
3+	Tonsils occupy 51%–75% of the lateral dimension of the oropharynx
4+	Tonsils occupy more than 75% of the lateral dimension of the oropharynx

enuresis, retardation of growth, behavioral and learning issues (hyperactivity, impulsivity, rebelliousness, aggression), and cardiovascular diseases (hypertension, cor pulmonale, ventricular dysfunction).[16]

The diagnosis of OSA in children is often made by history and physical examination with a positive predictive value of 50% to 60%.[17] When obtaining a history, parents may describe habitual snoring, restless sleep, mouth breathing, enuresis, diaphoresis, observed apnea, or sleep resistance behaviors. Overnight in-laboratory polysomnography (PSG) is considered "the gold standard" for the diagnosis of pediatric OSA.[17] This study allows for the diagnosis and assessment of disturbances in respiratory and sleep patterns, providing clinicians with objective data for the management of their patients. The apnea-hypopnea index (AHI) is the most commonly used parameter for quantifying the severity of OSA. This index represents the combined number of apneas and hypopneas that occur per hour of sleep. In the pediatric population, an AHI less than 1 is considered normal; > greater than >1 AHI ≤5 as mild OSA; > greater than 5 AHI ≤10 as moderate OSA; and greater than 10 as severe OSA. The clinical practice guideline from the American Academy of Otolaryngology – Head and Neck Surgery Society (AAO-HNS) recommends PSG in all cases for which the need for tonsillectomy is uncertain or when there is discordance between the physical examination and the reported severity of oSDB.[18] PSG is recommended for children less than 2 years of age as they are at higher risk of having postoperative respiratory complications. Children exhibiting the following should also undergo PSG as they are at risk for having residual OSA postoperatively: obesity, Down syndrome, craniofacial abnormalities, neuromuscular disorders, sickle cell disease, or mucopolysaccharidoses. Tonsillectomy and adenoidectomy is recommended for all children diagnosed with OSA as documented by PSG.[6]

Outcome data regarding adenotonsillectomy have been shown to improve PSG parameters, with a "cure rate" reported between 70% and 90%.[6,16] Disease-specific and global QOL measures have also been shown to be improved.[19] The Childhood Adenotonsillectomy Trial (CHAT), published in 2011, was a randomized controlled trial assessing the health and neurologic outcomes in children with OSA after adenotonsillectomy. This study found that surgery reduced symptoms of OSA and improved behavior, QOL, and polysomnographic findings. However, there was no significant improvement in attention or executive function after adenotonsillectomy.[20] Children with OSA and concurrent enuresis may also derive benefit from adenotonsillectomy. Basha and colleagues reported a marked improvement or resolution of enuresis in most children with OSA who underwent tonsillectomy or adenotonsillectomy.[21] Likewise, a systematic review by Lehmann and colleagues showed complete or partial resolution in a majority of children.[22]

A number of studies have demonstrated that a subset of patients may experience weight gain following tonsillectomy. Increased weight gainwas noted primarily in the first 6 months postoperatively and predominantly in obese children.[20,23–25] However, more recent studies dispute these findings. Kirkham and colleagues and Jensen and colleagues both performed repeat analysis of the initial CHAT study data and reported no undesirable weight gain over a 7 month period following adenotonsillectomy when comparing BMI Z-scores and BMI expressed as a percentage of the 95th percentile, respectively.[26,27]

Recurrent Tonsillitis

Current AAO-HNS guidelines recommend tonsillectomy for patients with recurrent tonsillitis at a frequency of at least 7 episodes in the past year; at least 5 episodes per year for 2 years; or at least 3 episodes per year for 3 years. Each of these episodes should have documentation of fever greater than 38C (101F), cervical lymphadenopathy, tonsillar exudate, or culture positive for GABHS.[6] These recommendations are based on the Paradise criteria, which are shown in **Table 2**. Tonsillectomy for less severe disease may be recommended in patients with antibiotic allergies or recurrent peritonsillar abscess. .

Outcome data for tonsillectomy in children with recurrent tonsillitis have demonstrated mixed benefits for recurrent pharyngitis episodes postoperatively. Two studies by Paradise and colleagues examined the benefits of tonsillectomy in patients with severe episodes (based on the author's own scoring system) and reported that frequency and severity of throat infections were significantly reduced for 2 years postoperatively.[28] A follow-up study examining patients with less severe cases showed only modest benefit postoperatively.[29] A follow-up Cochrane review of 5 pooled studies corroborated these studies and demonstrated 1 year of benefit as compared with watchful waiting, with severely affected children more likely to benefit.[4] However, improvement in QOL was shown to be significant following tonsillectomy for

Table 2 Paradise criteria for tonsillectomy	
Criteria	**Definition**
Minimum frequency of sore throat episodes	At least 7 episodes in the previous year, at least 5 episodes in each of the previous 2 years, or at least 3 episodes in each of the previous 3 years
Clinical features	Sore throat plus at least one of the following features qualifies as a counting episode: Temperature of >100.9°F (38.3°C) Cervical adenopathy (tender lymph nodes or lymph node size >2 cm) Tonsillar exudate Culture positive for group A β-hemolytic streptococcus
Treatment	Antibiotics administered in the conventional dosage for proved or suspected streptococcal episodes
Documentation	Each episode of throat infection and its qualifying features substantiated by contemporaneous notation in a medical record If the episodes are not fully documented, subsequent observance by the physician of 2 episodes of throat infection with patterns of frequency and clinical features consistent with the initial history
Indications for Adenoidectomy	
History	Four or greater episodes of recurrent purulent rhinorrhea within 12 mo in a child <12 y of age. One episode should be documented by intranasal examination or diagnostic imaging. Persisting symptoms of adenoiditis after 2 courses of antibiotic therapy. One course of antibiotics should be with a B-lactamase stable antibiotic for at least 2 weeks. Sleep disturbance with nasal airway obstruction persisting for at least 3 mo Otitis media with effusion >3 mo or associated with additional sets of tubes. Otitis media with effusion (age 4 or greater)
Physical Exam	Description of uvula, palate, tonsils, nasal airway, cervical lymph nodes. Evaluation of adenoids by mirror, nasal endoscopy, or imaging only as necessary.

all cases of recurrent tonsillitis. In a prospective observational study, clinically significant improvements were seen across all Tonsil and Adenoid Health Status instrument (TAHSI) categories including airway and breathing, recurrent infection, health care utilization, health care costs, eating and swallowing, and behavior at 6 months and 1 year after surgery.[5] Further QOL subsets such as health perception, physical functioning, parental impact, and family impact were found to be significantly improved as well. It is also important to note that general satisfaction with tonsillectomy was reported in 91% of parents and caregivers.[30] While benefits for recurrent pharyngitis episodes may be modest, improvement in QOL indicators has been shown to be significant following tonsillectomy. Clinicians and families should discuss these potential benefits and risks before proceeding with surgery.

Periodic Fever, Aphthous Stomatitis, Pharyngitis, and Cervical Adenitis

PFAPA is a condition that may be confused with recurrent infectious tonsillitis. PFAPA is an acronym for an idiopathic inflammatory syndrome of periodic fevers, adenitis, pharyngitis, and aphthous stomatitis, first described by Marshall in 1987.[31] The hallmark of PFAPA is recurrent high fever that occurs with "clockwork" regularity every 2 to 8 weeks. Greater than 90% of patients will have pharyngitis, 75% will have cervical adenitis and up to 50% will have aphthous stomatitis. Onset is usually before 6 years of age and resolution typically occurs 3 to 5 years after onset.[32] Even though PFAPA is a self-limited condition, there can be a significant disease burden from recurrent episodes. Oral steroids are effective in controlling the symptoms but may result in a shorter interval between episodes. Tonsillectomy has been found to be effective in producing remission in up to 98% of patients with PFAPA.[33–35] Therefore, in children, experiencing an adverse QOL as a result of PFAPA, tonsillectomy is a reasonable option for treatment.

Chronic Tonsillitis

Chronic tonsillitis is defined as sore throat or pharyngitis of at least 3 months' duration accompanied by tonsillar inflammation, often with improvement in symptoms with antibiotics but no resolution. Chronic tonsillitis is relatively uncommon and no evidence-based data is available for outcomes after tonsillectomy. Chronic tonsillitis may also be associated with halitosis. This condition can arise from multiple origins including periodontal disease, glossal debris, gastroesophageal disorders, foreign bodies, and sinusitis. Halitosis can occur when there is stagnation of saliva, build-up of food debris, and accumulation of bacteria, usually retained in the crypts of the tonsils.[36,37] While halitosis is often cited as an indication for surgery, there is currently insufficient evidence to support the use of adenotonsillectomy for management.

Peritonsillar Abscess

Peritonsillar abscess (PTA), also known as quinsy, occurs when a collection of pus fills the space between the tonsillar capsule and the pharyngeal constrictor muscles. Patients present with fever, dysphagia, odynophagia, trismus, and "hot potato" or muffled voice. Physical examination will reveal an erythematous and edematous soft palate withuvular deviation away from the infected side. Initial management consists of incision and drainage or needle aspiration paired with antibiotics and systemic steroids. Tonsillectomy should be considered in patients who have experienced greater than 1 PTA.[6] A low threshold for surgery should be kept for patients who develop PTA with a history of frequent tonsil disease. Quinsy tonsillectomy, in which surgery is performed in the setting of an active infection, is occasionally considered if a child requires general anesthesia for drainage.

Malignancy

Non-Hodgkin lymphoma accounts for the majority of pediatric tonsillar malignancies.[38] A high index of suspicion is appropriate in children who present with rapid unilateral tonsil enlargement, tonsillar asymmetry characterized as greater than 2 grades on the Brodsky scale, or concurrent prominent cervical lymphadenopathy, night sweats, and fevers.[38,39]

SURGICAL TECHNIQUE
History

Tonsillectomy is one of the oldest surgical procedures still in existence. A description of partial removal of the tonsils first appears in texts from ancient India in 1000 BC, with the author exhorting the practitioner to refrain from removing the entire tonsil for fear of fatal hemorrhage. Celsus described a technique for the complete removal of tonsils as early as 50 AD.[40] However, partial tonsillectomy remained the more widely used procedure until the latter part of the 19th century when Ballenger introduced the technique of extracapsular dissection of the tonsil.[40,41]

It was not until the early 20th century, with improvements in anesthesia and hemostasis that total tonsillectomy became widely accepted.

Total or extracapsular tonsillectomy is performed by identifying the tonsillar capsule and dissecting in the plane between the tonsillar capsule and the pharyngeal musculature, removing the tonsil in its entirety. Tonsillectomy is most commonly performed with monopolar electrocautery or bipolar radiofrequency ablation (coblation), although other techniques such as cold steel (knife or snare) dissection or harmonic scalpel are also in use.

Complications

Tonsillectomy is generally a safe procedure. It is important, however, to understand and recognize the potential complications related to this surgery. The most common serious complication of tonsillectomy is hemorrhage. Primary bleeding occurs within the first 24 hours of surgery and is rare with an estimated rate of less than 1%. Secondary bleeding usually occurs 7 to 10 days postoperatively at rates between 2% and 4%.[42–44] Older patients (>11 years of age) have been shown to bleed more often after surgery.[45]

Patients can expect to experience sore throat and otalgia postoperatively. Multiple studies have compared the effect of various techniques on postoperative pain with evidence supporting coblation for reduced postoperative pain as well as the time needed to return to normal diet and activity.[46,47] Patients may also experience otalgia—usually during the first postoperative week. This pain occurs via referred pain from the glossopharyngeal nerve rather than via Eustachian tube injury or edema as no relationship has been noted between throat pain, otalgia, and negative middle ear pressures.[48] Ibuprofen and acetaminophen have been shown to be safe and effective for pain control following adenotonsillectomy.[49] Opioids, specifically, codeine which has a black box warning, should be avoided for pediatric patients with OSAS.

Postoperative pain can result in decreased oral intake, leading to dehydration. Following hemorrhage, dehydration is the most common postoperative complication resulting in hospital admission. Admission for dehydration occurs in less than 1% of patients and when needed, admission is usually under 24 hours.[50]

Respiratory compromise should also be monitored following adenotonsillectomy. Complications can be classified as major and minor. Major complications include postoperative pulmonary edema, laryngospasm, and bronchospasm. Minor complications include apnea exacerbation and hypoxemia with the need for oxygen supplementation. Patients with congenital disorders, cerebral palsy, seizure disorders, prematurity, and age less than 3 years are more likely to have major respiratory complications.[51–53] and should be observed in a monitored setting postoperatively.

Tonsillectomy can be performed safely as a same day procedure.[54] The American Academy of Pediatrics and AAO-HNS suggest that patients with risk factors for postoperative complications be managed in an inpatient setting. These factors focus on patients with decreased respiratory reserve and include obesity, significant comorbidities, severe OSA, or patients younger than 3 years of age.[6,48,55] The AAO-HNS guidelines recommend overnight monitoring for all children under the age of 3 or those who have severe OSA (AHI >10 or oxygen saturation nadir <80%). Inpatient care should include pain control, continuous pulse oximetry, and fluid management with either PO intake or IV fluids.

Intracapsular tonsillectomy

Partial intracapsular tonsillectomy (IT) or tonsillotomy was reintroduced by Koltai in 2002.[56] In this procedure, tonsillar tissue is removed by a microdebrider or bipolar radiofrequency ablation (coblation) from within the tonsillar capsule. The tonsillar capsule and a small rim of residual tonsil tissue serve as a "biological dressing" protecting the neurovascular structures within the underlying muscle. A recent systematic review of pooled data showed that IT was superior to extracapsular total tonsillectomy with respect to postoperative pain, analgesic use, and time to resumption of normal diet and activity. Furthermore, the incidence of postoperative readmission for bleeding or dehydration was significantly decreased with IT.[57] Postoperative secondary bleeding rates have been reported to be less than 1% in 2 large series.[58,59] The disadvantage of IT, however, is that there is a risk of regrowth of the residual tonsil. The reoperation rate has been reported to be less than 1% to 3%.[58–60] Children less than 4 years of age at the time of IT may be at increased risk of regrowth.[61] This data supports the benefits of IT over extracapsular tonsillectomy with an acceptable low risk of reoperation. The AAO-HNS guidelines do not address IT as a treatment for OSA. However, there is a growing body of literature supporting the efficacy of IT in select patients with OSA.[62–64]

ADENOIDECTOMY

Adenoidectomy may be performed with or without tonsillectomy. The most common indication for this procedure is obstructive sleep-disordered breathing and OSA. As with tonsillar hypertrophy, adenoid hypertrophy causes nasopharyngeal narrowing leading to partial or complete obstruction, especially with the loss of neuromuscular tone during sleep. Other indications include chronic or recurrent otitis media with effusion (cOME), chronic rhinorrhea, nasal obstruction, sinusitis, and chronic adenoiditis.

Given the central location of the adenoids in the upper respiratory tract and the proximity to the eustachian tube, adenoid hypertrophy was hypothesized to cause physical obstruction of the Eustachian tubes and nasal cavity thereby preventing mucus drainage and leading to infection. Interestingly, studies have demonstrated that adenoidectomy reduces chronic OME symptoms regardless of the size of the adenoid pad.[65,66] Multiple studies have examined the bacterial load of the adenoid pad and found that the adenoid pad serves as a reservoir for bacteria to form biofilms rather than causing mechanical obstruction of the Eustachian tube.[67,68]

In 2014, Wallace and colleagues reported that adenoidectomy reduced OME and improved hearing as compared with either myringotomy or observation.[69] Further systematic reviews demonstrated that adenoidectomy reduced the number of days experienced with OME over a 12 month period and also decreased the rate of repeat tympanostomy tube placement in children greater than 4 years of age.[68,70] As a result of these studies, adenoidectomy is recommended by the AAO-HNS for children over 4 years of age with chronic OME or in children receiving their second set of tubes.

Pediatric recurrent rhinosinusitis is also thought to be related to adenoid biofilm formation. A study by Brietzke found a correlation of sinonasal-symptom scores with quantitative bacteriologic findings in the adenoid core and not with adenoid size.[71] Additionally, Coticchia and colleagues compared adenoid tissue removed for chronic rhinosinusitis versus oSDB and found a statistically significantly larger biofilm surface area in the tissue from the rhinosinusitis patients.[72] These authors concluded that recurrent sinusitis despite medical therapy is due to biofilms, and adenoidectomy is the best therapeutic option to mechanically disrupt and eradicate the biofilms. The AAO-HNS guidelines recommend adenoidectomy in children less than 12 years of age with at least 4 episodes of recurrent purulent rhinorrhea in 12 months with at least one episode documented by intranasal examination or diagnostic imaging.

Chronic adenoiditis involves adenoid inflammation with resultant nasal obstruction, snoring, mouth breathing, and persistent purulent rhinitis unresponsive to antibiotics. These symptoms are similar to the manifestations of adenoid hypertrophy and can easily lead to confusion between the 2 conditions. As with rhinosinusitis and cOME, the etiology of chronic adenoiditis stems from biofilm formation. No controlled trials have been established to help guide management. Adenoidectomy, however, can disrupt the biofilm and address the local obstruction and may be offered to patients who have failed medical management.

Surgical Technique

Adenoidectomy can be completed by a variety of techniques. Traditional excision is completed via loop adenoid curettes. The use of this technique is declining; however, as more clinicians have transitioned to microdebridement and electrosurgical devices. Electrocautery adenoidectomy provides the benefits of greater precision while also minimizing blood loss and reducing surgical time. Of note, it is important to understand that the adenoid is not an encapsulated structure like the tonsils, but rather fronds of tissue.[73] Thus, adenoidectomy never results in complete removal and tissue regrowth becomes a potential concern with regrowth rates reported between 1% and 9% and revision required in approximately 3% of cases.[74,75]

Complications

In general, adenoidectomy is well tolerated with low rates of complications. Velopharyngeal insufficiency (VPI) is a rare complication associated with adenoidectomy and manifests as hypernasal speech and nasal regurgitation. VPI has a reported incidence of 1 in 1500 and is more likely to occur in patients with hypotonia or submucosal cleft palate.[76,77] Nasopharyngeal stenosis or eustachian tube scarring may also occur as a result of excessive excision or electrocautery of the tonsillar pillars or posterior pharyngeal wall. Compared with tonsillectomy, adenoidectomy complications are infrequent and the procedure is associated with minmal postoperative pain, dehydration, postoperative bleeding, as well as shorter hospital stays, and lower cost.

SUMMARY

This article provides a brief overview of the indications, surgical techniques, and outcomes for adenoidectomy and tonsillectomy. Tonsillectomy should be performed in children with recurrent tonsillitis meeting the Paradise criteria, with oSDB or OSA, and in some cases of PTA, PFAPA, or concern for malignancy. Adenoidectomy is indicated in children with chronic otitis media with effusion, recurrent rhinosinusitis, and chronic adenoiditis.

CLINICS CARE POINTS

- Adenotonsillectomy has been shown to be effective in treating OSA with improvement in symptoms, behavior, and PSG and QOL measures postoperatively.
- Tonsillectomy for recurrent pharyngitis has modest benefits and in some cases, is no better than watchful waiting.
- Adentonsillectomy can be safely performed as an outpatient procedure in children greater than 3 years of age; children with significant comorbidities and severe OSA should be observed overnight postoperatively.
- Adenoidectomy is recommended in children greater than 4 years of age with chronic otitis media with effusion.
- Adenoidectomy is recommended for the treatment of recurrent sinusitis in children less than 12 years of age.

REFERENCES

1. Bohr C, Shermetaro C. Tonsillectomy and Adenoidectomy. In: StatPearls. Stat-Pearls Publishing; 2021. Available at: http://www.ncbi.nlm.nih.gov/books/NBK536942/. Accessed September 14, 2021.
2. Erickson BK, Larson DR, St Sauver JL, et al. Changes in incidence and indications of tonsillectomy and adenotonsillectomy, 1970-2005. Otolaryngol Head Neck Surg 2009;140(6):894–901.
3. Patel HH, Straight CE, Lehman EB, et al. Indications for tonsillectomy: a 10 year retrospective review. Int J Pediatr Otorhinolaryngol 2014;78(12):2151–5.
4. Burton MJ, Glasziou PP, Chong LY, et al. Tonsillectomy or adenotonsillectomy versus non-surgical treatment for chronic/recurrent acute tonsillitis. Cochrane Database Syst Rev 2014;11. https://doi.org/10.1002/14651858.CD001802.pub3.
5. Goldstein NA, Stewart MG, Witsell DL, et al. Quality of life after tonsillectomy in children with recurrent tonsillitis. Otolaryngol Head Neck Surg 2008;138(1 Suppl):S9–16.
6. Mitchell RB, Archer SM, Ishman SL, et al. Clinical practice guideline: tonsillectomy in children (update). Otolaryngol Head Neck Surg 2019;160(1_suppl):S1–42.
7. Isaacson G, Parikh T. Developmental anatomy of the tonsil and its implications for intracapsular tonsillectomy. Int J Pediatr Otorhinolaryngol 2008;72(1):89–96.
8. Goeringer GC, Vidić B. The embryogenesis and anatomy of Waldeyer's ring. Otolaryngol Clin North Am 1987;20(2):207–17.
9. Arambula A, Brown JR, Neff L. Anatomy and physiology of the palatine tonsils, adenoids, and lingual tonsils. World J Otorhinolaryngol Head Neck Surg 2021;7(3):155–60.
10. Jaw TS, Sheu RS, Liu GC, et al. Development of adenoids: a study by measurement with MR images. Kaohsiung J Med Sci 1999;15(1):12–8.
11. Handelman CS, Osborne G. Growth of the nasopharynx and adenoid development from one to eighteen years. Angle Orthodontist 1976;46(3):243–59.

12. Cahali MB, de Paula Soares CF, da Silva Dantas DA, et al. Tonsil volume, tonsil grade and obstructive sleep apnea: is there any meaningful correlation? Clinics (Sao Paulo) 2011;66(8):1347–51.

13. Marcus CL, Fernandes Do Prado LB, Lutz J, et al. Developmental changes in upper airway dynamics. J Appl Physiol (1985) 2004;97(1):98–108.

14. Dehlink E, Tan H-L. Update on paediatric obstructive sleep apnoea. J Thorac Dis 2016;8(2):224–35.

15. SAVINI S, CIORBA A, BIANCHINI C, et al. Assessment of obstructive sleep apnoea (OSA) in children: an update. Acta Otorhinolaryngol Ital 2019;39(5): 289–97.

16. Marcus CL, Brooks LJ, Ward SD, et al. Diagnosis and Management of Childhood Obstructive Sleep Apnea Syndrome. Pediatrics 2012;130(3):e714–55.

17. Brietzke SE, Katz ES, Roberson DW. Can history and physical examination reliably diagnose pediatric obstructive sleep apnea/hypopnea syndrome? A systematic review of the literature. Otolaryngol Head Neck Surg 2004;131(6):827–32.

18. Liu H, Feng X, Sun Y, et al. Modified adenoid grading system for evaluating adenoid size in children: a prospective validation study. Eur Arch Otorhinolaryngol 2021;278(6):2147–53.

19. Stewart MG, Glaze DG, Friedman EM, et al. Quality of life and sleep study findings after adenotonsillectomy in children with obstructive sleep apnea. Arch Otolaryngol Head Neck Surg 2005;131(4):308–14.

20. Redline S, Amin R, Beebe D, et al. The Childhood Adenotonsillectomy Trial (CHAT): Rationale, Design, and Challenges of a Randomized Controlled Trial Evaluating a Standard Surgical Procedure in a Pediatric Population. Sleep 2011;34(11):1509–17.

21. Basha S, Bialowas C, Ende K, et al. Effectiveness of adenotonsillectomy in the resolution of nocturnal enuresis secondary to obstructive sleep apnea. Laryngoscope 2005;115(6):1101–3.

22. Lehmann KJ, Nelson R, MacLellan D, et al. The role of adenotonsillectomy in the treatment of primary nocturnal enuresis in children: A systematic review. J Pediatr Urol 2018;14(1):53.e1-8.

23. Lewis TL, Johnson RF, Choi J, et al. Weight gain after adenotonsillectomy: a case control study. Otolaryngol Head Neck Surg 2015;152(4):734–9.

24. AlAbdullah ZA, Alali K, Al Jabr I. Clinical assessment of weight gain in pediatric patients post-tonsillectomy: a retrospective study. Cureus 2020;12(12):e12005.

25. Barr GS, Osborne J. Weight gain in children following tonsillectomy. J Laryngol Otol 1988;102(7):595–7.

26. Kirkham EM, Leis AM, Chervin RD. Weight gain in children after adenotonsillectomy: undesirable weight gain or catch-up growth? Sleep Med 2021;85:147–9.

27. Jensen AM, Herrmann BW, Mitchell RB, et al. Growth After Adenotonsillectomy for Obstructive Sleep Apnea: Revisited. Laryngoscope 2021. https://doi.org/10.1002/lary.29863.

28. Paradise JL, Bluestone CD, Bachman RZ, et al. Efficacy of Tonsillectomy for Recurrent Throat Infection in Severely Affected Children. N Engl J Med 1984; 310(11):674–83.

29. Paradise JL, Bluestone CD, Colborn DK, et al. Tonsillectomy and adenotonsillectomy for recurrent throat infection in moderately affected children. Pediatrics 2002;110(1 Pt 1):7–15.

30. Wolfensberger M, Haury JA, Linder T. Parent satisfaction 1 year after adenotonsillectomy of their children. Int J Pediatr Otorhinolaryngol 2000;56(3):199–205.

31. Marshall GS, Edwards KM, Butler J, et al. Syndrome of periodic fever, pharyngitis, and aphthous stomatitis. J Pediatr 1987;110(1):43–6.
32. Batu ED. Periodic fever, aphthous stomatitis, pharyngitis, and cervical adenitis (PFAPA) syndrome: main features and an algorithm for clinical practice. Rheumatol Int 2019;39(6):957–70.
33. Licameli G, Lawton M, Kenna M, et al. Long-term surgical outcomes of adenotonsillectomy for PFAPA syndrome. Arch Otolaryngol Head Neck Surg 2012;138(10): 902–6.
34. Lantto U, Koivunen P, Tapiainen T, et al. Long-Term Outcome of Classic and Incomplete PFAPA (Periodic Fever, Aphthous Stomatitis, Pharyngitis, and Adenitis) Syndrome after Tonsillectomy. J Pediatr 2016;179:172–7.e1.
35. Erdogan F, Kulak K, Öztürk O, et al. Surgery vs medical treatment in the management of PFAPA syndrome: a comparative trial. Paediatr Int Child Health 2016; 36(4):270–4.
36. Madhushankari GS, Yamunadevi A, Selvamani M, et al. Halitosis – An overview: Part-I – Classification, etiology, and pathophysiology of halitosis. J Pharm Bioallied Sci 2015;7(Suppl 2):S339–43.
37. Kapoor U, Sharma G, Juneja M, et al. Halitosis: Current concepts on etiology, diagnosis and management. Eur J Dent 2016;10(2):292–300.
38. Adil EA, Medina G, Cunningham MJ. Pediatric tonsil cancer: a national and institutional perspective. J Pediatr 2018;197:255–61.e1.
39. Berkowitz RG, Mahadevan M. Unilateral tonsillar enlargement and tonsillar lymphoma in children. Ann Otol Rhinol Laryngol 1999;108(9):876–9.
40. Grob GN. The rise and decline of tonsillectomy in twentieth-century America. J Hist Med Allied Sci 2007;62(4):383–421.
41. Verma R, Verma RR, Verma RR. Tonsillectomy-comparative study of various techniques and changing trend. Indian J Otolaryngol Head Neck Surg 2017;69(4): 549–58.
42. Krishna P, Lee D. Post-tonsillectomy bleeding: a meta-analysis. Laryngoscope 2001;111(8):1358–61.
43. Wall JJ, Tay K-Y. Postoperative Tonsillectomy Hemorrhage. Emerg Med Clin North Am 2018;36(2):415–26.
44. Dhaduk N, Rodgers A, Govindan A, et al. Post-Tonsillectomy Bleeding: A National Perspective. Ann Otol Rhinol Laryngol 2021;130(8):941–7.
45. Myssiorek D, Alvi A. Post-tonsillectomy hemorrhage: an assessment of risk factors. Int J Pediatr Otorhinolaryngol 1996;37(1):35–43.
46. Vieira L, Nissen L, Sela G, et al. Reducing postoperative pain from tonsillectomy using monopolar electrocautery by cooling the oropharynx. Int Arch Otorhinolaryngol 2014;18(2):155–8.
47. Omrani M, Barati B, Omidifar N, et al. Coblation versus traditional tonsillectomy: A double blind randomized controlled trial. J Res Med Sci 2012;17(1):45–50.
48. Randall DA. Current Indications for Tonsillectomy and Adenoidectomy. J Am Board Fam Med 2020;33(6):1025–30.
49. Diercks GR, Comins J, Bennett K, et al. Comparison of ibuprofen vs acetaminophen and severe bleeding risk after pediatric tonsillectomy: a noninferiority randomized clinical trial. JAMA Otolaryngol Head Neck Surg 2019;145(6):494–500.
50. Randall DA, Hoffer ME. Complications of tonsillectomy and adenoidectomy. Otolaryngol Head Neck Surg 1998;118(1):61–8.
51. Biavati MJ, Manning SC, Phillips DL. Predictive Factors for Respiratory Complications After Tonsillectomy and Adenoidectomy in Children. Arch Otolaryngol Head Neck Surg 1997;123(5):517–21.

52. Richmond KH, Wetmore RF, Baranak CC. Postoperative complications following tonsillectomy and adenoidectomy–who is at risk? Int J Pediatr Otorhinolaryngol 1987;13(2):117–24.

53. Marrugo Pardo G, Romero Moreno LF, Beltrán Erazo P, et al. Respiratory Complications of Adenotonsillectomy for Obstructive Sleep Apnea in the Pediatric Population. Sleep Disord 2018;2018:1968985.

54. Amoils M, Chang KW, Saynina O, et al. Postoperative Complications in Pediatric Tonsillectomy and Adenoidectomy in Ambulatory vs Inpatient Settings. JAMA Otolaryngol Head Neck Surg 2016;142(4):344–50.

55. Werle AH, Nicklaus PJ, Kirse DJ, et al. A retrospective study of tonsillectomy in the under 2-year-old child: indications, perioperative management, and complications. Int J Pediatr Otorhinolaryngol 2003;67(5):453–60.

56. Koltai PJ, Solares CA, Mascha EJ, et al. Intracapsular partial tonsillectomy for tonsillar hypertrophy in children. Laryngoscope 2002;112(8 Pt 2 Suppl 100):17–9.

57. Lee HS, Yoon HY, Jin HJ, et al. The safety and efficacy of powered intracapsular tonsillectomy in children: A meta-analysis. Laryngoscope 2018;128(3):732–44.

58. Soaper AL, Richardson ZL, Chen JL, et al. Pediatric tonsillectomy: A short-term and long-term comparison of intracapsular versus extracapsular techniques. Int J Pediatr Otorhinolaryngol 2020;133:109970.

59. Amin N, Bhargava E, Prentice JG, et al. Coblation intracapsular tonsillectomy in children: A prospective study of 1257 consecutive cases with long-term follow-up. Clin Otolaryngol 2021. https://doi.org/10.1111/coa.13790.

60. Sorin A, Bent JP, April MM, et al. Complications of microdebrider-assisted powered intracapsular tonsillectomy and adenoidectomy. Laryngoscope 2004; 114(2):297–300.

61. Sagheer SH, Kolb CM, Crippen MM, et al. Predictive Pediatric Characteristics for Revision Tonsillectomy After Intracapsular Tonsillectomy. Otolaryngol Head Neck Surg 2021. https://doi.org/10.1177/01945998211034454. 1945998211034454.

62. Chang DT, Zemek A, Koltai PJ. Comparison of treatment outcomes between intracapsular and total tonsillectomy for pediatric obstructive sleep apnea. Int J Pediatr Otorhinolaryngol 2016;91:15–8.

63. Mukhatiyar P, Nandalike K, Cohen HW, et al. Intracapsular and Extracapsular Tonsillectomy and Adenoidectomy in Pediatric Obstructive Sleep Apnea. JAMA Otolaryngol Head Neck Surg 2016;142(1):25–31.

64. Mostovych N, Holmes L, Ruszkay N, et al. Effectiveness of Powered Intracapsular Tonsillectomy in Children With Severe Obstructive Sleep Apnea. JAMA Otolaryngol Head Neck Surg 2016;142(2):150–6.

65. Saafan ME, Ibrahim WS, Tomoum MO. Role of adenoid biofilm in chronic otitis media with effusion in children. Eur Arch Otorhinolaryngol 2013;270(9):2417–25.

66. Bayazian G, Sayyahfar S, Safdarian M, et al. Is there any association between adenoid biofilm and upper airway infections in pediatric patients? Turk Pediatri Ars 2018;53(2):71–7.

67. Boonacker CW, Rovers MM, Browning GG, et al. Adenoidectomy with or without Grommets for Children with Otitis Media: An Individual Patient Data Meta-Analysis. Health Technol Assess 2014;18(5):1–118.

68. van den Aardweg MT, Schilder AG, Herkert E, et al. Adenoidectomy for otitis media in children. Cochrane Database Syst Rev 2010;1:CD007810.

69. Wallace IF, Berkman ND, Lohr KN, et al. Surgical treatments for otitis media with effusion: a systematic review. Pediatrics 2014;133(2):296–311.

70. Mikals SJ, Brigger MT. Adenoidectomy as an Adjuvant to Primary Tympanostomy Tube Placement: A Systematic Review and Meta-analysis. JAMA Otolaryngol Head Neck Surg 2014;140(2):95–101.
71. Brietzke SE, Shin JJ, Choi S, et al. Clinical Consensus Statement: Pediatric Chronic Rhinosinusitis. Otolaryngol Head Neck Surg 2014;151(4):542–53.
72. Coticchia J, Zuliani G, Coleman C, et al. Biofilm surface area in the pediatric nasopharynx: Chronic rhinosinusitis vs obstructive sleep apnea. Arch Otolaryngol Head Neck Surg 2007;133(2):110–4.
73. Dearking AC, Lahr BD, Kuchena A, et al. Factors associated with revision adenoidectomy. Otolaryngol Head Neck Surg 2012;146(6):984–90.
74. Babademez MA, Gul F, Muz E, et al. Impact of partial and total tonsillectomy on adenoid regrowth. Laryngoscope 2017;127(3):753–6.
75. Lesinskas E, Drigotas M. The incidence of adenoidal regrowth after adenoidectomy and its effect on persistent nasal symptoms. Eur Arch Otorhinolaryngol 2009;266(4):469–73.
76. Hubbard BA, Rice GB, Muzaffar AR. Adenoid involvement in velopharyngeal closure in children with cleft palate. Can J Plast Surg 2010;18(4):135–8.
77. Donnelly MJ. Hypernasality following adenoid removal. Ir J Med Sci 1994;163(5): 225–7.

Pediatric Obstructive Sleep Apnea

Update for the Primary Care Provider

Pakkay Ngai, MD[a], Michael Chee, MD[b],*

KEYWORDS

- Obstructive sleep apnea (OSA) • Pediatric • Polysomnography
- Adenotonsillectomy (AT)

KEY POINTS

- Obstructive sleep apnea (OSA) occurs commonly in children and if untreated, may lead to neurobehavioral and cardiovascular consequences.
- Polysomnography remains the gold standard for the diagnosis of OSA; however, availability may be limited and indications for performance of polysomnography have not reached a consensus.
- Adenotonsillectomy is the first-line treatment of OSA, although management options for mild OSA have expanded to include observation, weight loss, or medication therapy.
- Persistent OSA symptoms after tonsillectomy may be evaluated with polysomnography, sleep endoscopy, or cine MRI.

INTRODUCTION

Pediatric obstructive sleep apnea (OSA) syndrome is a disorder that is inadequately screened for, despite its prevalence of 1% to 4% in children.[1] Initially described in 1892 by Sir William Olser and then with a case series published in 1976,[2] pediatric OSA is characterized by cyclic episodes of partial (hypopnea) or complete (apnea) airway obstruction, or a pattern of obstructive hypoventilation consisting of periods of persistent partial upper airway obstruction associated with hypercapnia, arterial oxygen desaturation, or both.[3] Sleep pattern disruption may be observed. Although the physiologic derangements occur primarily during sleep, children with OSA may

Funding Sources: None.
Conflict of Interest: None.
[a] Division of Pediatric Pulmonology, Joseph M. Sanzari Children's Hospital, Hackensack Meridian Children's Health, 30 Prospect Avenue, WFAN 3rd Floor, Hackensack, NJ 07601, USA;
[b] Division of Pediatric Otolaryngology, Joseph M. Sanzari Children's Hospital, Hackensack Meridian Children's Health, 30 Prospect Avenue, WFAN PC-311, Hackensack, NJ 07601, USA
* Corresponding author.
E-mail address: michael.chee@hmhn.org

Pediatr Clin N Am 69 (2022) 261–274
https://doi.org/10.1016/j.pcl.2021.12.001
0031-3955/22/© 2022 Elsevier Inc. All rights reserved.

pediatric.theclinics.com

manifest both daytime and nighttime symptoms. When evaluating a child with sleep difficulties, the provider should recognize the interplay between medical and behavioral causes. Pediatric OSA represents a common medical sleep disorder that should be identified early. In this review, we explore the predisposing factors, diagnostic choices, and management strategies for pediatric OSA.

PREDISPOSING FACTORS

Although the pathophysiology of pediatric OSA is likely multifactorial, adenotonsillar hypertrophy is the most common cause.[4] In young children, enlargement of the adenoids and tonsils occurs frequently from ages 2 to 6 years. The adenoid and palatine tonsils both encroach upon the retropalatal area of the pharyngeal airway, leading to maximal narrowing where they overlap.[5,6] Tonsil size in children is typically described with the Brodsky scale, where the tonsils are assigned a grade from 1+ to 4+ according to the percentage of the oropharyngeal airway occupied by the tonsils.[7]

With the increase in its prevalence and severity, obesity has become an increasingly significant cause of pediatric sleep-disordered breathing, particularly among adolescents[8,9]; this is likely due to excessive fat deposition in areas of the pharyngeal airway, leading to decreased airway size and increased pharyngeal collapsibility.[10] Obesity increases the risk of persistent OSA after adenotonsillectomy.[6] Compared with normal-weight children, obese children benefited less from adenotonsillectomy,[11] with essentially no improvement in the polysomnography (PSG)-derived apnea-hypopnea index (AHI) in children classified with severe obesity (body mass index z score >3).[12]

Other associated medical conditions that have an increased prevalence of sleep-disordered breathing include Down syndrome, Prader-Willi syndrome, neuromuscular disorders (Duchenne muscular dystrophy), Chiari malformations, myelomeningocele, and craniofacial anomalies (achondroplasia, Pierre Robin sequence, craniofacial dysostosis).[13]

MORBIDITY

Signs and symptoms of pediatric OSA are reflected in nocturnal and diurnal manifestations. During any routine health care encounter, primary care providers should allow children and caretakers the opportunity to discuss their child's sleep habits and concerns.

Snoring is the most commonly observed symptom in pediatric sleep-disordered breathing, although many children who snore will not have OSA. Although it may be common to equate snoring with deep sleep, snoring is a sign of turbulent airflow causing the soft tissues to vibrate. However, even primary snoring, or snoring with the exclusion of OSA, has been associated with adverse neurocognitive consequences.[14,15] Other nocturnal signs and symptoms to note are mouth breathing, gasping, choking, and observed pauses in breathing. Pediatric OSA may also be associated with restless sleep, frequent awakenings, nocturnal diaphoresis, sleep enuresis, and increased frequency of parasomnia (sleep terrors, sleepwalking).

There are daytime consequences associated with pediatric OSA. Daytime sleepiness in children resulting from OSA is not as prevalent as in adult patients with OSA.[16] However, children with OSA may experience neurocognitive deficits and behavioral issues.[17,18] For children presenting with learning difficulties, poor school performance, hyperactivity, inattentiveness, impulsivity, disruptive behavior, or aggression, there is literature to support screening for sleep-disordered breathing.[18,19]

Although obesity is noted as a risk factor for OSA, younger children with OSA may conversely present with poor growth and weight gain,[20,21] likely due to the increased caloric expenditure caused by increased work of breathing during sleep.[20] Fortunately, with earlier recognition of OSA in infants and young children, failure to thrive status as a presenting feature of OSA is infrequently observed in this day and age, but should nonetheless be considered in the differential diagnosis of growth failure.[22]

Additional cardiovascular consequences arising from pediatric OSA include metabolic dysregulation, proinflammatory states, and oxidative stress. Independent of obesity, pediatric OSA leads to metabolic impairment with a greater risk of dyslipidemia, insulin resistance, and hypertension.[23] OSA in children has been linked with upregulation of a systemic inflammatory process caused by intermittent hypoxia and sleep fragmentation.[24] This intermittent hypoxia followed by recovery (reoxygenation) is thought to result in increased oxidative stress, with production of free radicals that have a role in the development and progression of cardiovascular disease in children with OSA.[25]

Pulmonary hypertension (PH) has been reported as a cardiovascular complication of pediatric OSA, which should be screened for in the setting of severe OSA.[17,26] However, a recent study found a low prevalence of PH in children with OSA. Of those patients with PH, none had severe OSA, suggesting that the severity of OSA may not accurately predict the risk of PH.[27]

DIAGNOSIS

In the third edition of the American Academy of Sleep Medicine's (AASM's) International Classification of Sleep Disorders, the diagnosis of pediatric OSA is met when 2 sets of criteria (A and B) are both met. Criterion A consists of (1) snoring; (2) labored, paradoxic, or obstructed breathing is observed; or (3) sleepiness, hyperactivity, behavioral or learning problems are noted. Criterion B focuses on PSG criteria. Either the patient experiences (1) one or more obstructive apneas, hypopneas, or mixed apneas per hour or (2) demonstrates a pattern of obstructive hypoventilation (greater than 25% of sleep time with $Paco_2$ >50 mm Hg), along with snoring, paradoxic thoracoabdominal motion (see-saw breathing), or a flattened inspiratory nasal pressure waveform.[3]

In practice, reaching this formal diagnosis of pediatric OSA will vary according to the available resources, namely, with respect to access to a pediatric sleep laboratory. Hence, there has been ongoing interest in developing validated measures to identify children at risk for sleep-disordered breathing and associated morbidities, particularly when the gold-standard test of nocturnal PSG is not obtainable. However, alternative diagnostic methods have been hindered by poorer positive and negative predictive outcomes relative to PSG. These methods have included home audio-video recording[28,29] pulse oximetry,[30,31] and questionnaires.[32] However, one widely used Pediatric Sleep Questionnaire[33] has been shown to predict postsurgical improvement among subjective measures of behavior, quality of life, and sleepiness, whereas PSG-derived severity of OSA was not predictive of neurobehavioral improvement.[34] Although there is widespread use of home sleep apnea testing in adults,[35] its usage is not recommended for the diagnosis of OSA in children after review by a 2017 AASM task force.[36]

Multichannel overnight in-laboratory PSG remains the gold-standard measure for the diagnosis of pediatric OSA.[13,37] Performance of a single-night PSG study has been demonstrated to be sufficient to assess for childhood sleep-disordered breathing.[38,39]

Acknowledging that access to sleep laboratories for children may be limited in parts of the country, there is debate about the widespread performance of PSG for all pediatric adenotonsillectomy candidates. A survey of pediatric otolaryngologists found that only 10% of children who underwent adenotonsillectomy had a preoperative PSG performed, with most cases decided by clinical diagnosis rather than PSG.[40] This decision making is at odds with the AASM[13] and American Academy of Pediatrics (AAP)[17] recommending PSG for all children undergoing tonsillectomy. The AAP does qualify that in circumstances when PSG is not readily available, it recommends referral to an otolaryngologist or a sleep medicine specialist.[17] In an update to the clinical practice guideline, the American Academy of Otolaryngology–Head and Neck Surgery (AAO-HNS) stands by the more limited use of PSG for children younger than 2 years, or with comorbidities including obesity, Down syndrome, craniofacial abnormalities, neuromuscular disorders, sickle cell disease, or mucopolysaccharidoses.[41,42]

When PSG is conducted, technical specifications for the performance and scoring of the study are detailed in the AASM Manual for the Scoring of Sleep and Associated Events.[43] Multiple variables are recorded, with attention to neurophysiologic and respiratory monitoring. Electroencephalography, electrooculography, and electromyography provide the data on which sleep staging (non–rapid eye movement [NREM]-1, NREM-2, NREM-3, REM) is determined. Electrocardiography, body position sensors, and audiovisual recording are standard components of PSG. Respiratory monitoring will involve oronasal airflow sensors, respiratory inductance plethysmography belts, pulse oximetry (oxygen saturation as measured by pulse oximetry), and capnometry (either end-tidal CO_2 or transcutaneous CO_2).[37] Measurement of these variables allows detection of events and the derivation of a summary report that is interpreted by a board-certified sleep medicine specialist.

In a child being evaluated for OSA, respiratory events (obstructive apnea, obstructive hypopnea, central apnea, or mixed apnea) are scored using pediatric scoring rules from updated versions of the AASM manual.[43] However, for adolescents between 13 and 18 years, respiratory scoring rules using adult criteria may instead be applied, at the discretion of the sleep specialist. Yet, it should be recognized that usage of adult standards may lead to an underestimation of respiratory events, given that the adult event duration requirement ($\geq$10 seconds) is longer than the pediatric criterion of 2 or more breath cycles.

Although the number of respiratory events per hour, known as the AHI, is tabulated from the PSG data, agreement upon the classification of the severity of pediatric OSA has not reached a consensus. A frequently used approach categorizes pediatric OSA into mild (AHI 1–5), moderate (AHI 5–10), or severe (AHI >10) degrees.[44] From the clinical practice guidelines of the AAO-HNS, severe OSA is regarded as an obstructive AHI $\geq$ 10 per hour or an oxygen saturation nadir less than 80%.[41,42]

TREATMENT/MANAGEMENT
Observation

Some clinicians advocate for observation of mild OSA in the absence of concerning findings on PSG or the lack of severe morbidity. Other clinicians advocate for observation of mild OSA because of its ephemeral nature. The 2013 CHAT [Childhood Adenotonsillectomy Trial] study[45] was a single-blind randomized controlled study comparing adenotonsillectomy with watchful waiting for the treatment of OSA in children aged 5 to 9. After the 7-month intervention period, the watchful waiting group had a 46% rate of resolution of OSA. The study result may have been affected by a small number of children who were also being treated with either a nasal steroid spray or montelukast (4%), but there remained a large cohort of children who improved without medical intervention. Sarber and colleagues[46] performed a retrospective chart review on children younger than 3 years with mild OSA and found that after an observation period between 3 and 12 months, 31% of patients had resolution of their condition.

Weight Loss

There is a growing body of evidence that weight loss may be an effective treatment of OSA in obese children. Anderson and colleagues[47] followed a group of obese children aged 7 to 18 during a 1-year enrollment in a multidisciplinary obesity treatment clinic. By the end of the study, they found that of the 62 children who were initially found to have OSA, 27 (44%) had resolution of their OSA. The reduction in body mass index standard deviation score was significantly associated with the reduction in AHI. There are also data from the bariatric literature showing that for the extremely obese, bariatric surgical intervention may lead to improvement in OSA.[48]

Medication

Over the years, clinicians have tried to use an array of medications for the treatment of pediatric OSA, some more successful than others. Al-Ghamdi and colleagues[49] performed a small open-label study looking at the effect of a 5-day course of oral prednisone on children with OSA and adenotonsillar hypertrophy. Only 1 in 9 children had enough improvement to avoid adenotonsillectomy. Topical nasal corticosteroids have been shown to reduce adenoid size and improve nasal congestion.[50] In vitro studies have shown that exposure to leukotriene antagonists leads to reduction in adenotonsillar cell proliferation.[51] A meta-analysis looked at the use of anti-inflammatory medications for the treatment of pediatric OSA. Five studies evaluated montelukast alone as a treatment of pediatric OSA and found a 55% mean decrease in AHI from 6.2 pretreatment to 2.8 posttreatment, with an improvement in lowest oxygen saturation from 89.5 to 92.1. Two studies evaluated the effects of both montelukast and intranasal corticosteroids on pediatric OSA and found a 70% mean decrease in AHI from 4.7 pretreatment to 1.4 posttreatment, with an improvement in mean lowest oxygen saturation from 87.8 to 92.6.[52] For mild OSA, a 12- to 16-week treatment course of intranasal steroids and montelukast seems to be beneficial. Although these medications are generally well tolerated, families should be counseled on the increased risk of depression and anxiety in adolescents.

Adenotonsillectomy

Adenotonsillectomy is a procedure in which both the palatine tonsils and the adenoids are completely removed. Multiple medical societies recommend adenotonsillectomy as one of the first-line treatments for pediatric OSA.[17,42] Although many techniques are available to complete the procedure no one specific technique has been recommended above others among these practice guidelines. Brietzke[53] performed a meta-analysis looking at the effectiveness of adenotonsillectomy for pediatric OSA. He found that the success rate of adenotonsillectomy for children without significant comorbidity was 82.9%. The 2013 CHAT[45] study showed that for children with OSA, adenotonsillectomy improved daytime symptoms of OSA, behavioral outcomes, and quality of life. The same study showed resolution of OSA in 79% of participants after adenotonsillectomy. This result also came after the exclusion of children with very severe OSA, severe hypoxia, and severe obesity. Costa and Mitchell[54] performed a meta-analysis looking at adenotonsillectomy for obese children with OSA. The investigators found that adenotonsillectomy in this population improves, but does not resolve OSA most of the time. Only 12% of children had a postoperative AHI less than 1. Other studies have shown significantly decreased effectiveness of adenoton-sillectomy for pediatric OSA in younger children and in those with severe OSA.[55]

Morbidity

Adenotonsillectomy is a surgical procedure that has both minor risks of pain and dehydration, as well as major risks, such as bleeding, postobstructive pulmonary edema, velopharyngeal insufficiency, and nasopharyngeal stenosis. The risk of postoperative bleeding seems to be similar, between 3% and 5%, among the various techniques used for adenotonsillectomy.[56] A study looking at the Kids' Inpatient Database showed that the children who had postoperative bleeding after adenotonsillectomy tended to be older and male.[57] Younger children, children with severe OSA, and children with craniofacial disorders seem to be more prone to postoperative respiratory compromise after adenotonsillectomy.[58]

Intracapsular Tonsillectomy and Adenoidectomy

Intracapsular tonsillectomy has been developed as an alternative to traditional extracapsular tonsillectomy. The procedure involves removing most of the tonsillar tissue while leaving a thin layer of tonsillar tissue in the tonsillar fossa. The technique theoretically reduces damage to the underlying muscular and neurovascular structures and in doing so, potentially reduces complication rates. A Cochrane review compared intracapsular versus extracapsular adenotonsillectomy for children with OSA. Both groups seem to have similar outcomes in terms of OSA resolution. The investigators found that postoperative pain was similar between the 2 groups, but that children who underwent intracapsular tonsillectomy and adenoidectomy (ITA) seemed to be able to return to normal activity more quickly (by 4 days). Complications that required medical or surgical intervention were also slightly better in the ITA group (2.6% vs 4.9%).[59] Unique risks attributable to ITA are the possibility of infection of the tonsillar remnant and tonsillar regrowth. The risk for tonsillar regrowth seems to be between 0.5% and 6% and can happen over the course of several years.[60,61]

Perioperative Monitoring

In children undergoing adenotonsillectomy for OSA, age and severity of OSA are associated with increased risk of postoperative respiratory complications. Children younger than 3 years or having severe OSA are recommended to be observed overnight after adenotonsillectomy. Postoperative care should incorporate continuous pulse oximetry and the availability of more intensive levels of care, including respiratory support.[42]

Persistent Obstructive Sleep Apnea after Adenotonsillectomy

Residual OSA is found in about 20% of children after adenotonsillectomy. The risk is even higher in children with severe OSA, obesity, craniofacial syndromes, and neuromuscular diseases.[53] For children who exhibit symptoms of persistent sleep disordered breathing 2 to 3 months after adenotonsillectomy, we recommend polysomnographic evaluation. Additional imaging modalities may also be considered in determining the site of obstruction.

Sleep Endoscopy

Drug-induced sleep endoscopy (DISE) is an examination of the upper airway using flexible endoscopy while the subject is sedated, but spontaneously breathing. Studies have shown that when a person sleeps, new and different sites of pharyngeal obstruction can emerge.[62] DISE has been shown to affect clinical decision making in children even before adenotonsillectomy has been performed.[63] Multiple studies have shown the utility of DISE in children with persistent OSA after adenotonsillectomy to identify sites of pharyngeal obstruction.[64,65] Although most clinicians who treat pediatric OSA believe that DISE is a helpful tool, there is substantial practice variation in how the procedure is performed and how the results are interpreted.[66] An expert consensus statement was formulated and advised that DISE would be helpful in cases of pediatric OSA with no tonsillar hypertrophy, children at high risk for persistent OSA after adenotonsillectomy, and in cases of persistent OSA after adenotonsillectomy.[67]

Cine MRI

Cine MRI has also been used to evaluate for sites of obstruction in children with OSA. Similarly to DISE, the evaluation is performed while the patient is sedated. The strength of cine MRI is its ability to dynamically evaluate the airway while looking at multiple sites at the same time. Several studies have shown good sensitivity and safety of the procedure.[68,69]

Continuous Positive Airway Pressure

Continuous positive airway pressure (PAP) is a therapeutic option in moderate-to-severe OSA cases where adenotonsillar hypertrophy is minimal/absent or when surgery is contraindicated or declined. Furthermore, with the upsurge in obesity, there has been increasing treatment with PAP for OSA that persists after adenotonsillectomy. Although PAP therapy is able to ameliorate the respiratory and sleep derangements of sleep-disordered breathing, its usage is also associated with neurobehavioral improvement in attention deficits, objective sleepiness, behavior, and quality-of-life measures.[70] However, the effectiveness of PAP is often offset by poor adherence. Children who are older, have less severe sleep-disordered breathing, or have less sleep disruption are more likely to be nonadherent to PAP therapy.[71] Enlisting family support and coaching is vital to the success of PAP, because lower maternal education was a strong predictor of poor PAP adherence.[72]

Nasal Surgery

Common causes of nasal congestion that may contribute to persistent OSA after adenotonsillectomy are turbinate hypertrophy, septal deviation, and adenoid regrowth. If medical therapy has inadequately treated turbinate hypertrophy, then turbinate reduction surgery is available and has been shown to improve OSA.[73] Septoplasty is usually reserved for patients who are at least 18 years old, due to observations of retarded nasal growth after septoplasty at a young age. The adult literature has shown some benefit of septoplasty for OSA, but this is usually in combination with other interventions. The regrowth rate of the adenoids after adenoidectomy is around 8%, but clinically significant cases are much less (2%). Adenoid regrowth can occur over the course of years.[74] In children with small tonsils, adenoidectomy alone has been shown to be an effective treatment of pediatric OSA.[75]

Oral Appliances

Oral appliances are mouthpieces that push the jaw and tongue forward, to create a larger airway and improve airflow during sleep. In children with retrognathia, another aim of the treatment is to redirect growth of the mandible into a more forward position. These should be considered for children who have mild to moderate OSA, had surgery that did not work, have difficulty using CPAP, and are not overweight. These devices are typically fit by dentists and orthodontists.[76]

Rapid Maxillary Expansion

Rapid maxillary expansion (RME) involves placing an expandable brace on the roof of the mouth that increases the width of the maxilla; this can be considered in children with high-arched and/or narrow hard palates (transverse maxillary deficiency). These devices are also typically fit by dentists and orthodontists. The ideal age of treatment is between 4 and 10 years. The use of RME has been shown to be helpful for mild pediatric OSA.[77]

Uvulopalatopharyngoplasty

Uvulopalatopharyngoplasty involves the removal and rearrangement of excessive uvular, palatal, and pharyngeal tissue. In adults, this procedure has been demonstrated to produce moderate benefit in the treatment of OSA. In pediatrics, this procedure has mostly been described for use in neurologically impaired patients leading to some benefit.[78,79]

Lingual Tonsillectomy

The lingual tonsils are a collection of lymphoid tissue on the dorsal surface of the tongue, between the circumvallate papillae and the root of the tongue. Lingual tonsil hypertrophy is often the site of obstruction for children with residual OSA after adenotonsillectomy, especially in children with Down syndrome. A meta-analysis examining the effectiveness of lingual tonsillectomy in persistent OSA showed that the procedure led to a mean change in reduction of AHI and an increase of minimum oxygen saturation of −6.64 and 4.17, respectively.[80]

Base of Tongue Surgery

Glossoptosis is defined as posterior motion of the tongue during sleep. As prolapse of the base of the tongue is often cited as a reason for persistent OSA after adenotonsillectomy,[81] several techniques have been developed to address this problem. Posterior midline glossectomy is performed by making a midline wedge resection on the posterior surface of the tongue and widening the oropharyngeal airway. Propst and colleagues[82] looked at children with Down syndrome and persistent OSA after tonsillectomy. Patients identified to have relative macroglossia underwent posterior midline glossectomy. Postoperatively, the AHI decreased from 47 to 5.6 for normal-weight individuals.

Tongue or hyoid suspension procedures work by using sutures to suspend the base of tongue with titanium screws placed into the lower mandible. Hypoglossal nerve stimulators are implanted devices that electrically stimulate the hypoglossal nerve, which causes tongue movement. The stimulation is timed with breathing to relieve upper airway obstruction. Suspension procedures and hypoglossal stimulation are techniques used mostly in adults, with little available data on pediatric patients. Hartzell and colleagues[83] looked at children with cerebral palsy and OSA, noting that patients with glossoptosis seemed to benefit from tongue base suspension procedures. Caloway and colleagues[84] examined a group of nonobese children with Down syndrome with persistent OSA after adenotonsillectomy who underwent hypoglossal nerve stimulation. The investigators found a median reduction in AHI by 85% and a median nightly usage of the device for 9.2 hours.

Mandibular advancement surgeries, which include mandibular distraction osteogenesis and mandibular advancement, address the issue of micrognathia. Mandibular distraction osteogenesis, which is typically performed in infants, involves making an incision in the mandible and slowly separating the split pieces while new bone forms in between. Mandibular advancement, which is typically performed in teenagers and adults, involves repositioning the jaw to relieve airway obstruction in a single stage. A meta-analysis of mandibular advancement surgeries for pediatric OSA demonstrated a reduction in AHI from a mean of 41.1 to 4.5.[85]

Laryngotracheal Surgery

Supraglottoplasty is a procedure that treats laryngomalacia. Laryngomalacia is a condition in which floppy tissue of the larynx falls into the airway during inspiration causing obstruction. Laryngomalacia has been identified as a common site of obstruction for children with persistent OSA after adenotonsillectomy. A review of studies looking at supraglottoplasty for pediatric OSA showed a resolution rate of OSA ranging from 58% to 72%.[68]

Tracheostomy is a procedure that creates an opening into the trachea in which a tube is placed. It is the definitive surgery for the treatment of upper airway obstruction. This procedure is usually reserved for cases of severe OSA for which other courses of treatment have failed and other types of surgery will not likely succeed.

SUMMARY

Pediatric OSA is a common entity that can cause both daytime and nighttime issues. Children with symptoms should be screened for OSA. If possible, PSG should be performed to evaluate symptomatic children. Depending on the severity, first-line options for treatment of pediatric OSA may include observation, weight loss, medication, or surgery. Even after adenotonsillectomy, about 20% of children will have persistent OSA. Sleep endoscopy and cine MRI are tools that may be used to identify sites of obstruction, which in turn can help in the selection of site-specific treatment.

CLINICS CARE POINTS

- The diagnosis and treatment of pediatric OSA can benefit from a multidisciplinary team approach.
- Although adenotonsillectomy is an effective treatment of OSA, clinicians should monitor for persistent OSA, which can warrant further investigation with PSG, sleep endoscopy, or cine MRI.

DISCLOSURE

Nothing to disclose.

REFERENCES

1. Lumeng JC, Chervin RD. Epidemiology of pediatric obstructive sleep apnea. Proc Am Thorac Soc 2008;5(2):242–52.
2. Guilleminault C, Eldridge FL, Simmons FB, et al. Sleep apnea in eight children. Pediatrics 1976;58(1):23–30.
3. American Academy of Sleep Medicine. International classification of sleep disorders. 3rd edition. Darien: AASM; 2014.
4. Brennan LC, Kirkham FJ, Gavlak JC. Sleep-disordered breathing and comorbidities: role of the upper airway and craniofacial skeleton. Nat Sci Sleep 2020;12: 907–36.

5. Arens R, Marcus CL. Pathophysiology of upper airway obstruction: a developmental perspective. Sleep 2004;27(5):997–1019.

6. Gulotta G, Iannella G, Vicini C, et al. Risk factors for obstructive sleep apnea syndrome in children: state of the art. Int J Environ Res Public Health 2019;16(18):3235.

7. Brodsky L. Modern assessment of tonsils and adenoids. Pediatr Clin North Am 1989;36(6):1551–69.

8. Hannon TS, Rofey DL, Ryan CM, et al. Relationships among obstructive sleep apnea, anthropometric measures, and neurocognitive functioning in adolescents with severe obesity. J Pediatr 2012;160(5):732–5.

9. Spilsbury JC, Storfer-Isser A, Rosen CL, et al. Remission and incidence of obstructive sleep apnea from middle childhood to late adolescence. Sleep 2015;38(1):23–9.

10. Isono S. Obesity and obstructive sleep apnoea: mechanisms for increased collapsibility of the passive pharyngeal airway. Respirology 2012;17(1):32–42.

11. Andersen IG, Holm JC, Homøe P. Obstructive sleep apnea in obese children and adolescents, treatment methods and outcome of treatment - A systematic review. Int J Pediatr Otorhinolaryngol 2016;87:190–7.

12. Lennon CJ, Wang RY, Wallace A, et al. Risk of failure of adenotonsillectomy for obstructive sleep apnea in obese pediatric patients. Int J Pediatr Otorhinolaryngol 2017;92:7–10.

13. Aurora RN, Zak RS, Karippot A, et al. Practice parameters for the respiratory indications for polysomnography in children. Sleep 2011;34(3):379–88.

14. O'Brien LM, Gozal D. Behavioural and neurocognitive implications of snoring and obstructive sleep apnoea in children: facts and theory. Paediatr Respir Rev 2002;3(1):3–9.

15. Hagström K, Saarenpää-Heikkilä O, Himanen SL, et al. Neurobehavioral Outcomes in School-Aged Children with Primary Snoring. Arch Clin Neuropsychol 2020;35(4):401–12.

16. Gozal D, Wang M, Pope DW Jr. Objective sleepiness measures in pediatric obstructive sleep apnea. Pediatrics 2001;108(3):693–7.

17. Marcus CL, Brooks LJ, Draper KA, et al. Diagnosis and management of childhood obstructive sleep apnea syndrome. Pediatrics 2012;130(3):e714–55.

18. Trosman I, Trosman SJ. Cognitive and behavioral consequences of sleep disordered breathing in children. Med Sci (Basel) 2017;5(4):30.

19. Hunter SJ, Gozal D, Smith DL, et al. Effect of sleep-disordered breathing severity on cognitive performance measures in a large community cohort of young school-aged children. Am J Respir Crit Care Med 2016;194(6):739–47.

20. Marcus CL, Carroll JL, Koerner CB, et al. Determinants of growth in children with the obstructive sleep apnea syndrome. J Pediatr 1994;125(4):556–62.

21. Freezer NJ, Bucens IK, Robertson CF. Obstructive sleep apnoea presenting as failure to thrive in infancy. J Paediatr Child Health 1995;31(3):172–5.

22. Esteller E, Villatoro JC, Agüero A, et al. Obstructive sleep apnea syndrome and growth failure. Int J Pediatr Otorhinolaryngol 2018;108:214–8.

23. Patinkin ZW, Feinn R, Santos M. Metabolic consequences of obstructive sleep apnea in adolescents with obesity: a systematic literature review and meta-analysis. Child Obes 2017;13(2):102–10.

24. Gozal D. Sleep, sleep disorders and inflammation in children. Sleep Med 2009;10(Suppl 1):S12–6.

25. Doğruer ZN, Unal M, Eskandari G, et al. Malondialdehyde and antioxidant enzymes in children with obstructive adenotonsillar hypertrophy. Clin Biochem 2004;37(8):718–21.
26. Ingram DG, Singh AV, Ehsan Z, et al. Obstructive sleep apnea and pulmonary hypertension in children. Paediatr Respir Rev 2017;23:33–9.
27. Burns AT, Hansen SL, Turner ZS, et al. Prevalence of pulmonary hypertension in pediatric patients with obstructive sleep apnea and a cardiology evaluation: a retrospective analysis. J Clin Sleep Med 2019;15(8):1081–7.
28. Sivan Y, Kornecki A, Schonfeld T. Screening obstructive sleep apnoea syndrome by home videotape recording in children. Eur Respir J 1996;9(10):2127–31.
29. Lamm C, Mandeli J, Kattan M. Evaluation of home audiotapes as an abbreviated test for obstructive sleep apnea syndrome (OSAS) in children. Pediatr Pulmonol 1999;27(4):267–72.
30. Brouillette RT, Morielli A, Leimanis A, et al. Nocturnal pulse oximetry as an abbreviated testing modality for pediatric obstructive sleep apnea. Pediatrics 2000; 105(2):405–12.
31. Hornero R, Kheirandish-Gozal L, Gutiérrez-Tobal GC, et al. Nocturnal oximetry-based evaluation of habitually snoring children. Am J Respir Crit Care Med 2017;196(12):1591–8.
32. Patel AP, Meghji S, Phillips JS. Accuracy of clinical scoring tools for the diagnosis of pediatric obstructive sleep apnea. Laryngoscope 2020;130(4):1034–43.
33. Chervin RD, Hedger K, Dillon JE, et al. Pediatric sleep questionnaire (PSQ): validity and reliability of scales for sleep-disordered breathing, snoring, sleepiness, and behavioral problems. Sleep Med 2000;1(1):21–32.
34. Rosen CL, Wang R, Taylor HG, et al. Utility of symptoms to predict treatment outcomes in obstructive sleep apnea syndrome. Pediatrics 2015;135(3):e662–71 [published correction appears in Pediatrics. 2016 Apr;137(4):].
35. Kapur VK, Auckley DH, Chowdhuri S, et al. Clinical Practice Guideline for Diagnostic Testing for Adult Obstructive Sleep Apnea: An American Academy of Sleep Medicine Clinical Practice Guideline. J Clin Sleep Med 2017;13(3): 479–504.
36. Kirk V, Baughn J, D'Andrea L, et al. American Academy of Sleep Medicine position paper for the use of a home sleep apnea test for the diagnosis of OSA in children. J Clin Sleep Med 2017;13(10):1199–203.
37. Stowe RC, Afolabi-Brown O. Pediatric polysomnography-A review of indications, technical aspects, and interpretation. Paediatr Respir Rev 2020;34:9–17.
38. Katz ES, Greene MG, Carson KA, et al. Night-to-night variability of polysomnography in children with suspected obstructive sleep apnea. J Pediatr 2002;140(5): 589–94.
39. Li AM, Wing YK, Cheung A, et al. Is a 2-night polysomnographic study necessary in childhood sleep-related disordered breathing? Chest 2004;126(5):1467–72.
40. Mitchell RB, Pereira KD, Friedman NR. Sleep-disordered breathing in children: survey of current practice. Laryngoscope 2006;116(6):956–8.
41. Roland PS, Rosenfeld RM, Brooks LJ, et al. Clinical practice guideline: Polysomnography for sleep-disordered breathing prior to tonsillectomy in children. Otolaryngol Head Neck Surg 2011;145(1 Suppl):S1–15.
42. Mitchell RB, Archer SM, Ishman SL, et al. Clinical practice guideline: tonsillectomy in children (update). Otolaryngol Head Neck Surg 2019;160(1_suppl): S1–42.
43. Berry RB, Quan SF, Abreu AR, et al, for the American Academy of Sleep Medicine. The AASM manual for the scoring of sleep and associated events: rules,

terminology and technical specifications, version 2.6. Darien (IL): American Academy of Sleep Medicine; 2020.

44. Katz ES, Marcus CL. Diagnosis of obstructive sleep apnea syndrome in infants and children. In: Sheldon SH, Ferber R, Kryger MH, editors. Principles and practice of pediatric sleep medicine. Elsevier Saunders; 2005. p. 197–210.

45. Marcus CL, Moore RH, Rosen CL, et al. Childhood Adenotonsillectomy Trial (CHAT). A randomized trial of adenotonsillectomy for childhood sleep apnea. N Engl J Med 2013;368(25):2366–76.

46. Sarber KM, von Allmen DC, Tikhtman R, et al. Polysomnographic outcomes after observation for mild obstructive sleep apnea in children younger than 3 years. Otolaryngol Head Neck Surg 2021;164(2):427–32.

47. Andersen IG, Holm JC, Homøe P. Impact of weight-loss management on children and adolescents with obesity and obstructive sleep apnea. Int J Pediatr Otorhinolaryngol 2019;123:57–62.

48. Kalra M, Inge T, Garcia V, et al. Obstructive sleep apnea in extremely overweight adolescents undergoing bariatric surgery. Obes Res 2005;13(7):1175–9.

49. Al-Ghamdi SA, Manoukian JJ, Morielli A, et al. Do systemic corticosteroids effectively treat obstructive sleep apnea secondary to adenotonsillar hypertrophy? Laryngoscope 1997;107(10):1382–7.

50. Demain JG, Goetz DW. Pediatric adenoidal hypertrophy and nasal airway obstruction: reduction with aqueous nasal beclomethasone. Pediatrics 1995; 95(3):355–64.

51. Dayyat E, Serpero LD, Kheirandish-Gozal L, et al. Leukotriene pathways and in vitro adenotonsillar cell proliferation in children with obstructive sleep apnea. Chest 2009;135(5):1142–9.

52. Liming BJ, Ryan M, Mack D, et al. Montelukast and nasal corticosteroids to treat pediatric obstructive sleep apnea: a systematic review and meta-analysis. Otolaryngol Head Neck Surg 2019;160(4):594–602.

53. Brietzke SE, Gallagher D. The effectiveness of tonsillectomy and adenoidectomy in the treatment of pediatric obstructive sleep apnea/hypopnea syndrome: a meta-analysis. Otolaryngol Head Neck Surg 2006;134(6):979–84.

54. Costa DJ, Mitchell R. Adenotonsillectomy for obstructive sleep apnea in obese children: a meta-analysis. Otolaryngol Head Neck Surg 2009;140(4):455–60.

55. Friedman M, Wilson M, Lin HC, et al. Updated systematic review of tonsillectomy and adenoidectomy for treatment of pediatric obstructive sleep apnea/hypopnea syndrome. Otolaryngol Head Neck Surg 2009;140(6):800–8.

56. Pynnonen M, Brinkmeier JV, Thorne MC, et al. Coblation versus other surgical techniques for tonsillectomy. Cochrane Database Syst Rev 2017;8(8):CD004619.

57. Dhaduk N, Rodgers A, Govindan A, et al. Post-tonsillectomy bleeding: a national perspective. Ann Otol Rhinol Laryngol 2021;130(8):941–7.

58. McColley SA, April MM, Carroll JL, et al. Respiratory Compromise After Adenotonsillectomy in Children With Obstructive Sleep Apnea. Arch Otolaryngol Head Neck Surg 1992;118(9):940–3.

59. Blackshaw H, Springford LR, Zhang L-Y, et al. Tonsillectomy versus tonsillotomy for obstructive sleep-disordered breathing in children. Cochrane Database Syst Rev 2020;(4):CD011365.

60. Solares CA, Koempel JA, Hirose K, et al. Safety and efficacy of powered intracapsular tonsillectomy in children: a multi-center retrospective case series. Int J Pediatr Otorhinolaryngol 2005;69(1):21–6.

61. Windfuhr JP, Savva K, Dahm JD, et al. Tonsillotomy: facts and fiction. Eur Arch Otorhinolaryngol 2015;272(4):949–69.

62. Soares D, Folbe AJ, Yoo G, et al. Drug-induced sleep endoscopy vs awake Müller's maneuver in the diagnosis of severe upper airway obstruction. Otolaryngol Head Neck Surg 2013;148(1):151–6.

63. Boudewyns A, Saldien V, Van de Heyning P, et al. Drug-induced sedation endoscopy in surgically naïve infants and children with obstructive sleep apnea: impact on treatment decision and outcome. Sleep Breath 2018;22(2):503–10.

64. Socarras MA, Landau BP, Durr ML. Diagnostic techniques and surgical outcomes for persistent pediatric obstructive sleep apnea after adenotonsillectomy: A systematic review and meta-analysis. Int J Pediatr Otorhinolaryngol 2019;121: 179–87.

65. Coutras SW, Limjuco A, Davis KE, et al. Sleep endoscopy findings in children with persistent obstructive sleep apnea after adenotonsillectomy. Int J Pediatr Otorhinolaryngol 2018;107:190–3.

66. Friedman NR, Parikh SR, Ishman SL, et al. The current state of pediatric drug-induced sleep endoscopy. Laryngoscope 2017;127(1):266–72.

67. Baldassari CM, Lam DJ, Ishman SL, et al. Expert consensus statement: pediatric drug-induced sleep endoscopy. Otolaryngol Head Neck Surg 2021;165(4): 578–91.

68. Manickam PV, Shott SR, Boss EF, et al. Systematic review of site of obstruction identification and non-CPAP treatment options for children with persistent pediatric obstructive sleep apnea. Laryngoscope 2016;126(2):491–500.

69. Isaiah A, Kiss E, Olomu P, et al. Characterization of upper airway obstruction using cine MRI in children with residual obstructive sleep apnea after adenotonsillectomy. Sleep Med 2018;50:79–86.

70. Marcus CL, Radcliffe J, Konstantinopoulou S, et al. Effects of positive airway pressure therapy on neurobehavioral outcomes in children with obstructive sleep apnea. Am J Respir Crit Care Med 2012;185(9):998–1003.

71. Blinder H, Momoli F, Holland SH, et al. Clinical predictors of nonadherence to positive airway pressure therapy in children: a retrospective cohort study. J Clin Sleep Med 2021;17(6):1183–92.

72. DiFeo N, Meltzer LJ, Beck SE, et al. Predictors of positive airway pressure therapy adherence in children: a prospective study. J Clin Sleep Med 2012;8(3):279–86.

73. Cheng PW, Fang KM, Su HW, et al. Improved objective outcomes and quality of life after adenotonsillectomy with inferior turbinate reduction in pediatric obstructive sleep apnea with inferior turbinate hypertrophy. Laryngoscope 2012;122(12): 2850–4.

74. Paramaesvaran S, Ahmadzada S, Eslick GD. Incidence and potential risk factors for adenoid regrowth and revision adenoidectomy: A meta-analysis [published correction appears in Int J Pediatr Otorhinolaryngol. 2021 Oct;149:110885]. Int J Pediatr Otorhinolaryngol 2020;137:110220.

75. Domany KA, Dana E, Tauman R, et al. Adenoidectomy for obstructive sleep apnea in children. J Clin Sleep Med 2016;12(9):1285–91.

76. Yanyan M, Min Y, Xuemei G. Mandibular advancement appliances for the treatment of obstructive sleep apnea in children: a systematic review and meta-analysis. Sleep Med 2019;60:145–51.

77. Camacho M, Chang ET, Song SA, et al. Rapid maxillary expansion for pediatric obstructive sleep apnea: A systematic review and meta-analysis. Laryngoscope 2017;127(7):1712–9.

78. Kerschner JE, Lynch JB, Kleiner H, et al. Uvulopalatopharyngoplasty with tonsillectomy and adenoidectomy as a treatment for obstructive sleep apnea in neurologically impaired children. Int J Pediatr Otorhinolaryngol 2002;62(3):229–35.

79. Kosko JR, Derkay CS. Uvulopalatopharyngoplasty: treatment of obstructive sleep apnea in neurologically impaired pediatric patients. Int J Pediatr Otorhinolaryngol 1995;32(3):241–6.
80. Rivero A, Durr M. Lingual tonsillectomy for pediatric persistent obstructive sleep apnea: a systematic review and meta-analysis. Otolaryngol Head Neck Surg 2017;157(6):940–7.
81. Raposo D, Menezes M, Rito J, et al. Drug-induced sleep endoscopy in pediatric obstructive sleep apnea. Otolaryngol Head Neck Surg 2021;164(2):414–21.
82. Propst EJ, Amin R, Talwar N, et al. Midline posterior glossectomy and lingual tonsillectomy in obese and nonobese children with down syndrome: Biomarkers for success. Laryngoscope 2017;127(3):757–63.
83. Hartzell LD, Guillory RM, Munson PD, et al. Tongue base suspension in children with cerebral palsy and obstructive sleep apnea. Int J Pediatr Otorhinolaryngol 2013;77(4):534–7.
84. Caloway CL, Diercks GR, Keamy D, et al. Update on hypoglossal nerve stimulation in children with down syndrome and obstructive sleep apnea. Laryngoscope 2020;130(4):E263–7.
85. Noller MW, Guilleminault C, Gouveia CJ, et al. Mandibular advancement for pediatric obstructive sleep apnea: A systematic review and meta-analysis. J Craniomaxillofac Surg 2018;46(8):1296–302.

Pediatric Rhinosinusitis

Hassan H. Ramadan, MD, MSc[a],*, Rafka Chaiban, MD[b],
Chadi Makary, MD[a]

KEYWORDS

- Rhinosinusitis • Pediatrics • Sinus surgery • Endoscopic sinus surgery

KEY POINTS

- Definition and diagnosis of rhinosinusitis in children.
- Workup, differential diagnosis, and medical management of pediatric rhinosinusitis.
- Surgical options for rhinosinusitis in children, including adenoidectomy, balloon sinuplasty, and endoscopic sinus surgery (ESS).

BACKGROUND

Rhinosinusitis is a common diagnosis that is encountered by providers of all disciplines. Pediatric acute rhinosinusitis (ARS) and chronic rhinosinusitis (CRS) account for up to 2% of the total annual visits to the outpatient clinics and emergency departments[1]; they consume a large portion of the health care expenditure in the United States.[1] One of the challenges when dealing with pediatric rhinosinusitis is to make the correct diagnosis. Symptoms are usually like those of other conditions that include common cold, allergic rhinitis, and adenoiditis. Once correct diagnosis is made, appropriate treatment measures can be initiated. Younger children may have different presenting symptoms when compared with older ones. Cough and colored discharge are the main presenting symptoms for the young, whereas nasal stuffiness and facial pressure/headache will be the main ones in older children. It is important to recognize rhinosinusitis in children due to the potential serious complications and impact it may have on quality of life of those children.[2,3] Medical management is the mainstay of treatment, and, fortunately, it is successful in most of those children. When medical management fails, or a complication occurs, surgery may be required.

DEFINITIONS

Rhinosinusitis is an inflammation of the nose and paranasal sinuses; it is classified based on duration of symptoms. Acute rhinosinusitis (ARS) is when symptoms resolve

[a] Department of Otolaryngology–Head and Neck Surgery, West Virginia University, Morgantown, WV, USA; [b] Department of Pediatrics, West Virginia University, Uniontown, PA, USA
* Corresponding author. One Medical Center Drive, PO Box 9200. Morgantown, WV. 26506-9200
E-mail address: hramadan@hsc.wvu.edu

Pediatr Clin N Am 69 (2022) 275–286
https://doi.org/10.1016/j.pcl.2022.01.002
0031-3955/22/© 2022 Elsevier Inc. All rights reserved.

in less than 4 weeks, whereas CRS is when symptoms last for more than 12 weeks. Recurrent acute rhinosinusitis is defined as 4 or more episodes of ARS per year with resolution of symptoms between episodes.[2,3]

ACUTE RHINOSINUSITIS

ARS is defined as the onset of 2 or more of the following symptoms: nasal blockage/obstruction/congestion, discolored nasal discharge, or cough (daytime and nighttime) for less than 12 weeks.[2,3] ARS can theoretically be divided into acute viral rhinosinusitis (common cold), postviral rhinosinusitis, and acute bacterial rhinosinusitis.[4] One of the biggest challenges for clinicians is distinguishing ARS from a viral upper respiratory tract infection (URI). Data suggest that a child will average 6 to 8 episodes of the common cold in a season, and 1% to 5% of those URIs will develop into a sinus infection.[5] For an uncomplicated URI, symptoms start to resolve in 7 to 12 days. If the illness persists beyond 10 days or worsens after an initial improvement (double sickening), ARS is suspected.[2,3] ARS can be suspected from the initial onset of disease if 2 or more of the following signs and/or symptoms are present: discolored nasal discharge with unilateral predominance, purulent secretions, severe local pain with unilateral predominance, fever (>38°C), elevated erythrocyte sedimentation rate/C-reactive protein level.[3] *Streptococcus pneumoniae*, *Hemophilus influenzae,* and *Moraxella catarrhalis* are the most frequent bacteria in rhinosinusitis. Allergic rhinitis is another entity that can have similar symptoms to ARS, which make the diagnosis of ARS more challenging. It is important to take a good history as well as perform a comprehensive nasal examination with nasal endoscopy if possible.

Physical examination will include anterior rhinoscopy using a large speculum on an otoscope. Often, findings are nonspecific and include mucosal edema, inferior turbinate hypertrophy, and nasal drainage, which can be clear or thick-colored drainage. Examination of the throat may show purulent postnasal drainage.

Radiographic imaging is not indicated unless complications of ARS are suspected. Computed tomography (CT) of sinuses shows mucosal inflammation and opacification of the paranasal sinuses involved.

TREATMENT OF ACUTE RHINOSINUSITIS

For children with uncomplicated ARS, symptomatic treatment is recommended in the first 10 days given the likelihood of viral cause.[6] Oral antibiotics are recommended for patients with severe onset or worsening of the disease,[2,3] or if symptoms persist beyond 10 days. According to the American Academy of Pediatrics guidelines published in 2013, first-line empirical antibiotics treatment of ARS is amoxicillin without or with clavulanate.[7] Standard dosage should be considered unless there is a high risk for penicillin-resistant S pneumoniae. In that situation, high dose of amoxicillin clavulanate, defined as 90 mg/kg/d orally twice daily, should be used as a first-line therapy.[6,7] Second- or third-generation cephalosporins can be offered for patients with penicillin allergy. Duration of antibiotic treatment can vary anywhere from 10 to 20 days. In addition of oral antibiotics, intranasal saline sprays and intranasal corticosteroid sprays (INCS) should also be considered as adjunct treatments.[2,3]

COMPLICATIONS OF ACUTE RHINOSINUSITIS

Severe ARS can lead to several complications in children, and they can be classified as orbital, intracranial, and osseous complications. Orbital complications are the most common (60%–75%) and are classified based on Chandler's classification (**Table 1**),

Table 1
Chandler's classification of complications of acute rhinosinusitis

Chandler Class	Complication	Description
I	Preseptal cellulitis	Inflammation and edema of the eyelid anterior to the orbital septum
II	Orbital cellulitis	Inflammation extending into the orbital contents, posterior to the septum
III	Subperiosteal abscess	Abscess formation between the orbit bone and periorbita
IV	Orbital abscess	Abscess formation inside the orbital contents
V	Cavernous sinus thrombosis	Extension into the cavernous sinus causing ophthalmic deficits

which can range from preseptal cellulitis to cavernous sinus thrombosis.[8] Intracranial complications can include epidural, subdural, and/or brain abscess; meningitis; cerebritis; as well as superior sagittal and/or cavernous sinus thrombosis. Osseous complications include osteomyelitis of the frontal and maxillary bones. CT scan of the head and sinuses should be obtained as soon as complicated ARS is suspected (**Fig. 1**). CT has high accuracy to detect early orbital complications. MRI can be also considered and may be more sensitive for intracranial complications.

Early orbital complications can be managed medically with systemic antibiotic therapy with close follow-up for any clinical worsening.[9] Emergent surgical treatment is often needed in more advanced and severe complications, and when systemic antibiotic treatment alone fails.[8] Functional endoscopic sinus surgery (FESS) is often the surgical treatment of choice. Anterior orbitotomy is often needed to drain large orbital abscesses. A multidisciplinary team approach (otolaryngology, ophthalmology, neurosurgery, and infectious disease) is often required in these situations.

CHRONIC RHINOSINUSITIS

Pediatric CRS is defined as the presence of 2 or more of the following cardinal symptoms lasting for 12 weeks or longer: nasal obstruction, nasal discharge (anterior or posterior), facial pain/pressure, and cough.[2,3] Symptoms must be accompanied by objective evidence of inflammation, demonstrated on anterior rhinoscopy, nasal endoscopy, or radiography.[2,3]

Pediatric CRS is common in the United States, and it is diagnosed in up to 2.1% of pediatric patients in an ambulatory clinic setting per year.[1] In the United States alone, more than $1.8 billion is spent on treating CRS in children younger than 12 years annually.[1] CRS may start as a childhood viral URI initially, but up to 13% of these patients may have symptoms that progress to a chronic disease. A family history of CRS significantly increases the incidence of CRS diagnosis in children.[10]

Clinical symptoms of nasal discharge and cough are common in the young child. These symptoms can be URI, allergic rhinitis, adenoiditis, and/or rhinosinusitis. URI symptoms should be self-limiting, whereas allergy symptoms can be controlled with allergy medications. Adenoiditis/rhinosinusitis can have similar symptoms. Medical management is essentially the same. Differentiating between the 2 entities is important if condition becomes a surgical one, especially in the young child. Older children will present more commonly as their adult counterpart, with nasal congestion and facial

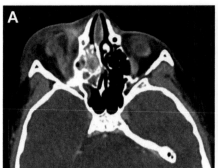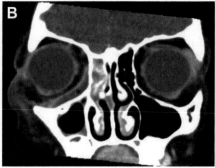

Fig. 1. CT scan soft tissue window axial cuts (*A*) and coronal cuts (*B*) of an 8-year-old boy who presented with rapidly progressing right eye swelling and proptosis. Large subperiosteal abscess can be appreciated (*asterisks*). Patient was taken emergently for surgical drainage of the abscess through an endoscopic approach.

pressure/pain. The adenoids would have regressed and will rarely be the cause of the symptoms.

CAUSE AND PATHOGENESIS

The cause of CRS is a subject of much debate and ongoing research. The pathogenesis is not fully elucidated, but it is likely to include multiple factors contributing to a complex disease entity. Several factors can contribute to the development of CRS.

The paranasal sinuses are a group of paired, aerated cavities that drain into the nasal cavity via the sinus ostia. Several ostia drain in the middle meatus leading to the "osteomeatal complex" as the focus of pathology.[11] Although the true anatomic role of the paranasal sinuses is uncertain, their ability to clear normal mucous secretions depends on 3 major factors: ostial patency, ciliary function, and mucous consistency.[12,13] Any variety of inciting factors may irritate the sinus mucosa leading to inflammation, edema, bacterial proliferation, outflow obstruction, and mucociliary dysfunction.

The association between CRS and allergic rhinitis has been well studied but continues to be controversial. There have been studies that showed that children with CRS have the same incidence of allergic rhinitis as in the general population, whereas other studies showed the opposite. Some studies also have shown that patients with perennial or seasonal allergic rhinitis had more significant radiographic findings of sinus disease.[14,15] Furthermore, patients with CRS with concomitant allergic rhinitis have a significantly decreased rate of long-term success following surgical treatment.[16]

Microbes have a controversial role in pediatric CRS. Although viral infections are known to precede episodes of viral rhinosinusitis,[17] viral infections are not usually targeted as a part of CRS treatment. The use of antibacterial agents, however, has remained a first-line treatment for many practitioners despite the questionable role of bacteria. The paranasal sinuses, normally considered sterile, house a characteristic set of bacteria in CRS. A recent study showed that greater than half of patients with CRS studied produced polymicrobial flora. The most common pathogens were those found in ARS. *Staphylococcus aureus* and coagulase-negative staphylococci were noted in those cultures from children with chronic disease as well. Anaerobes have been shown to be present in higher percentage in children with CRS.[18] The literature is replete with studies showing favorable patient response to treatment with antibiotics targeting these species, suggesting that there is some role for bacterial infection in CRS etiology.[19]

The role of inflammatory mediators in the pathogenesis of CRS in children is still vague. In adults, emphasis is made on inflammatory response to the presence of bacteria rather than the action of microbes themselves. The finding of a sinus mucosal infiltrate of eosinophils, plasma cells, and lymphocytes suggests a process of "bacterial allergy." There is likely a spectrum of illness ranging from an infectious etiology to a purely noninfectious inflammation.[20]

In children with asthma and CRS, it is important to treat CRS and have it well controlled, which leads to better asthma control.

Systemic factors can predispose to the development of CRS. Cystic fibrosis (CF) is an autosomal recessive disease that affects the upper and lower airways. Patients with CF nearly always develop chronic mucosal inflammation and nasal polyposis causing mechanical obstruction of sinus ostia.[21] Those patients are refractory to treatment and require multidisciplinary care including surgical treatment and topical therapies. Children who present with nasal polyps should always be tested for CF via a sweat chloride test and/or genetic testing.

Primary ciliary dyskinesia (PCD), although uncommon, is another systemic factor that can cause CRS. It is an autosomal recessive disorder caused by a defect in a specific element of mucociliary clearance.[22] A diagnosis of PCD should be considered in cases of refractory CRS, especially when accompanied with chronic and recurrent otitis media. PCD is often associated with situs inversus and bronchiectasis, known as Kartagener syndrome.

Other systemic factors that increase the risk of CRS in children is primary immunodeficiency disorders (PID). The true incidence of PID in patients with CRS is not known. Examples of PID include common variable immunodeficiency, Ig subclass deficiency, selective IgA deficiency, and specific antibody deficiency.

The role of gastroesophageal reflux disease (GERD) in pediatric CRS is still controversial and not very well studied. Expert opinion published recently agreed that routine treatment of GERD as part of CRS treatment is not needed. If treatment is necessary, it will have to be for the GERD symptoms and not for rhinosinusitis.[2,3,23]

When clinically suspected, testing for the presence of allergy or any of the other aforementioned conditions will assist in tailoring a treatment regimen.

DIFFERENTIAL DIAGNOSIS
Chronic Rhinosinusitis Versus Chronic Adenoiditis

Children with chronic symptoms of nasal stuffiness, discharge, and cough can have chronic adenoiditis, CRS, or both. Making the correct diagnosis based on symptoms alone can be extremely challenging. Medical treatment of both is essentially the same. The challenge is when medical treatment fails and surgical intervention is entertained. Nasal endoscopic examination, which may not be feasible in all children, can be helpful. However, in most instances, CRS can be present with chronic adenoiditis. Plain radiographs have poor specificity and sensitivity in diagnosing CRS and fail to correspond to the CT scan findings in up to 75% of the patients.[24] CT scan is the only gold standard in identifying the presence of CRS. It is extremely important that CT scan of the sinuses (**Fig. 2**) is performed at the end of appropriate maximal medical management. Once the scan is obtained, scoring the scan using a validated instrument, basically the Lund-McKay (LM) scoring system (**Table 2**) will allow for making the diagnosis. The scoring system consists of scoring each sinus of the 10 sinuses (5 on each side) with a zero if it completely clear, 1 if it is partially clear, and 2 if it

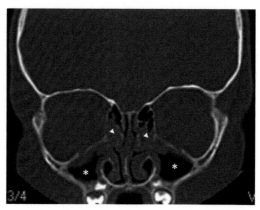

Fig. 2. CT scan sinuses bone window coronal cuts of a 4-year-old girl who failed appropriate medical therapy. Note the relatively small size of the maxillary sinuses (*asterisks*). Frontal sinuses are undeveloped, which is normal for this age group. Also note the mucosal thickening of the sinuses and blockage of the osteomeatal complexes (*arrowheads*).

completely opacified. Maxillary ostium blockage will be scored in addition to the rest of the sinuses on each side as well. It will be scored 0 if it is completely open and 2 if it is partially/completely opacified. Score will range from 0 to 24.[25] Bhattacharyya and colleagues[26] in a 2004 publication reviewed 66 children with symptoms of sinusitis/adenoiditis and compared them with 192 control patients. All patients had a CT scan of their sinuses. Upon using a CT Lund score of 5, they demonstrated that children with a CT score of 5 or higher exhibited true sinusitis with a sensitivity of 86% and specificity of 85%.[26] An LM CT score of less than 5 will thus denote chronic adenoiditis without sinusitis in the presence of symptoms. MRI has minimal role in diagnosis of pediatric CRS, and it is usually reserved in cases when complications or tumors are suspected.[2,3]

MEDICAL MANAGEMENT

The goal of medical management is to reduce sinonasal symptoms and reduce the inflammatory burden, and restoring the normal function of the sinuses. Oral antibiotics are the mainstay of treatment of CRS in children according to the most recent 2020

Table 2
Lund-McKay Computed tomography scoring system

Lund-Mackay CT Score	Right	Left
Maxillary sinus	0–2	0–2
Osteomeatal complex[a]	0 or 2	0 or 2
Anterior ethmoid sinus	0–2	0–2
Posterior ethmoid sinus	0–2	0–2
Sphenoid sinus	0–2	0–2
Frontal sinus	0–2	0–2
Total	0–12	0–12

0, no inflammation; 1, partial inflammation; 2, complete inflammation.
[a] 0, No obstruction; 1, obstructed.

European Position Paper on Rhinosinusitis & Nasal Polyps (EPOS) practice guidelines, the most extensive review on subject.[3] High-dose amoxicillin or amoxicillin-clavulanic acid are recommended as first line of treatment. Cephalosporins (second or third generations) or macrolides can be used as a second line of treatment or for those with penicillin allergy. There is no consensus on the duration of treatment, but most agree that it should be at least 3 weeks. Antibiotics can be repeated depending on the response of the child. Adjunct treatment consists of topical nasal saline sprays as well as INCS. Nasal saline sprays have shown to be effective in several studies[27]; they have shown to improve mucous clearance, enhance ciliary beat activity, and improve clearance of allergens and other mediators.[28] However, adherence and compliance are not well studied and are controversial.[29] INCS such as fluticasone and mometasone are safe and effective as first line or adjunct treatment in CRS with and without nasal polyps in children.[3] The addition of short courses of systemic corticosteroids has been shown to be effective in select patients. Short courses are usually used to treat inflammatory disorders of the sinuses unresponsive to INCS. However, the potential for serious side effects should limit the use of systemic corticosteroids for patients who are recalcitrant to conservative treatment.[30]

The role of intravenous antibiotics for the treatment of children with persistent or recurrent symptoms despite oral antibiotic management is not recommended for the treatment of uncomplicated CRS.[23] Parenteral antibiotics did not seem to contribute to a lasting resolution of children with CRS. The role of intravenous antibiotics in children is mainly for complicated rhinosinusitis. The role of GERD in the pathophysiology of CRS in children remains to be uncertain.[31] The role of reflux treatment in these children is equally unclear and based on recent guidelines is still not indicated.[23] Antibiotic prophylaxis to prevent infection in children who have recurrent episodes is also controversial. Little support is expressed for this approach based on other models, because of concerns of increasing prevalence of antibiotic-resistant organisms. Antibiotic prophylaxis may be used in patients with CF, PID, and PCD.[32]

It should be routine practice, that children with CRS be tested for immune deficiencies and referred to an immunologist. Recent review of our pediatric patients with CRS with PID showed intravenous immunoglobulin to be an effective treatment option for these patients.[33]

SURGICAL MANAGEMENT

Surgery for pediatric CRS has evolved significantly over the last 30 years. Surgery is reserved for children who have failed medical therapy. At present, endoscopic sinus surgery (ESS) is an accepted surgical treatment for both adults and children.[2,3,23] In adult population, ESS is the first-line surgical option resorted to for the treatment of CRS. In children, however, there are other surgical options to be considered other than ESS. Based on recent guidelines from EPOS 2020 and the 2014 American Academy of Otolaryngology (AAO) consensus statement adenoidectomy, sinus lavage, balloon dilation, and ESS are surgical treatments that have been used over the last 30 years.[3,23] Complicated sinusitis, fungal sinusitis, and nasal polyps are usually treated with ESS.[34] For CRS without complications, nasal polyposis, or fungal sinusitis, which surgical approach to use and when to operate remain somewhat unclear.

ADENOIDECTOMY

It is at present accepted that children who fail medical management as described earlier may require surgical intervention. Over the last 20 years, adenoidectomy has been proved to be successful in 50% to 71% of the patients and is recommended as first-line surgical treatment.[35,36] Because of the average success rate with adenoidectomy alone, a sinus wash at the time of adenoidectomy has been advocated, as an option before proceeding to FESS.[37] The procedure consists of flushing the sinuses, and at the same time a culture for antibiotic guidance would be obtained. Success rates with this procedure were noted to be around 88%. When reviewing the evidence, it is noted that adenoidectomy alone for patients with CRS, based on CT score, and in the presence of asthma, was not as successful; only 28% did well. Makary and Ramadan in 2014, reviewed 234 patients who had adenoidectomy only over a 10-year period; they divided patients into those with CRS (defined as CT LM score of 5 and more) and ones with chronic adenoiditis (CT score <5) based on Bhattacharya and colleagues[26] publication in 2004 that was discussed earlier. Retrospectively looking at success of CRS versus chronic adenoiditis, and using asthma as a comorbidity, the investigators found that adenoidectomy was successful in 28% of patients with CRS and asthma versus 71% for those who had chronic adenoiditis and no asthma (**Table 3**). Of note, older children (6 years and older) did not seem to do well with adenoidectomy alone.[38] Adenoidectomy seems to be helpful for younger kids, and for those with chronic adenoiditis without CRS (CT score <5) and no asthma with success rate of 71%.

BALLOON CATHETER SINUPLASTY

Balloon catheter sinuplasty (BCS) is another surgical treatment that can be considered for pediatric CRS. BCS can be used at the time of adenoidectomy or ESS as surgical adjunct to dilate the ostia as well as lavage the sinuses (**Fig. 3**). Prospective studies have shown that BCS is safe with minimal complications reported. Several publications have demonstrated that when BCS of the maxillary sinuses was performed at time of adenoidectomy, children had a better success rate than those who had adenoidectomy alone, 87% versus 54%.[39] The long-term efficacy of BCS still remains to be determined with larger prospective studies, even though recent studies have shown that success rate remained high 3 to 5 years postdilation.[40]

FUNCTIONAL ENDOSCOPIC SINUS SURGERY

FESS is a term used for minimally invasive procedures designed to restore the natural drainage pathways of the paranasal sinuses.[41] FESS is performed under general anesthesia, typically as a same-day procedure. The nasal cavity is directly visualized, and various specialized tools are used to relieve obstructive lesions of sinus outflow including polyps and diseased mucosa. The affected sinus air cells are opened in a

Table 3
Surgical success of adenoidectomy in chronic rhinosinusitis versus chronic adenoiditis

Variable	CRS	Chronic Adenoiditis	P Value
Patients	127 (57%)	97 (43%)	.52
Male sex	80 (63%)	57 (59%)	.75
Mean age	5	6.4	.0001
Allergy	56 (48%)	45 (51%)	.68
Asthma	53 (43%)	39 (42%)	.77
Success	54 (43%)	54 (65%)	.0017

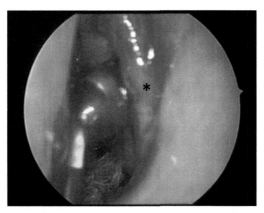

Fig. 3. Balloon catheter sinuplasty for the left maxillary sinus. Balloon is introduced behind the uncinate process (*asterisk*) into the natural ostium of the sinus.

manner that augments natural mucociliary outflow. ESS is now an accepted surgical treatment of pediatric CRS.[2,3,23] Otolaryngologists were initially reluctant to proceed with ESS, due to several factors that included fear of major complications in children as well as the fear of facial growth retardation.[42] Even though one study showed no difference in facial growth 10 years after ESS in children compared with a comparative group of children who had no surgery, that concern is still present.[43] In a 2013 systematic review, Makary and Ramadan[44] reviewed the literature between 1990 and 2012. After selecting only 11 studies that met the inclusion criteria out of 507 publications, they reported that ESS had success rates of more than 82% with a major complication rate of 1.4%. A similar systematic review and meta-analysis performed by Vlatarakos and colleagues,[45] also in 2013, reported a surgical success from 71% to 100% for improvement of Pediatric Chronic Rhinosinusitis (PCRS) symptoms and quality of life with a low incidence (0.6%) of major complications. At present, ESS is considered

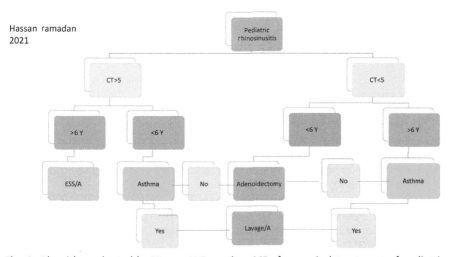

Fig. 4. Algorithm adapted by Hassan H Ramadan, MD, for surgical treatment of pediatric rhinosinusitis. A, adenoidectomy.

one of the main surgical options for certain children who meet strict criteria as defined by EPOS and AAO consensus statements.[2,3,23]

SUMMARY

Pediatric rhinosinusitis is a common disease in children. Knowledge of the evidence available for medical as well as surgical treatment can help significantly in the management of those children. There is significant consensus over medical management, and recently it seems that evidence for surgical management is becoming clearer. Making the diagnosis of CRS versus chronic adenoiditis is of utmost importance for surgical management. Adenoidectomy for younger children, with no asthma and with chronic adenoiditis without sinusitis, provides an excellent first-line surgical option. For older children, with CRS and asthma, sinus lavage/ESS seems to provide a better outcome for those children. An algorithm that we developed over the years is attached, which, we hope, may help clinicians in clinical decision making for surgical options when treating CRS in children (**Fig. 4**).

REFERENCES

1. Gilani S, Shin JJ. The burden and visit prevalence of pediatric chronic rhinosinusitis. Otolaryngol Head Neck Surg 2017;157(6):1048–52.
2. Fokkens WJ, Lund VJ, Hopkins C, et al. European Position Paper on Rhinosinusitis and Nasal Polyps 2020. Rhinology 2020;58(Suppl S29):1–464.
3. Orlandi RR, Kingdom TT, Smith TL, et al. International consensus statement on allergy and rhinology: rhinosinusitis 2021. Int Forum Allergy Rhinol 2021;11(3):213–739.
4. Brook I. Acute sinusitis in children. Pediatr Clin North Am 2013;60:409–24.
5. Revai K, Dobbs LA, Nair S, et al. Incidence of acute otitis media and sinusitis complicating upper respiratory tract infection: the effect of age. Pediatrics 2007;119:e1408–12.
6. Chow AW, Benninger MS, Brook I, et al. IDSA clinical practice guideline for acute bacterial rhinosinusitis in children and adults. Clin Infect Dis 2012;54(8):e72–112.
7. Wald ER, Applegate KE, Bordley C, et al. Clinical practice guideline for the diagnosis and management of acute bacterial sinusitis in children aged 1 to 18 years. Pediatrics 2013;132(1):e262–80.
8. Chandler JR, Langenbrunner DJ, Stevens ER. The pathogenesis of orbital complications in acute sinusitis. Laryngoscope 1970;80(9):1414–28.
9. Wong SJ, Levi J. Management of pediatric orbital cellulitis: A systematic review. Int J Pediatr Otorhinolaryngol 2018;110:123–9.
10. Orb Q, Curtin K, Oakley GM, et al. Familial risk of pediatric chronic rhinosinusitis. Laryngoscope 2016;126(3):739–45.
11. Lalwani AK. Current diagnosis & treatment in otolaryngology-head & neck surgery. 2nd edition. McGraw-Hill; 2008.
12. Lanza DC, Kennedy DW. Adult rhinosinusitis defined. Otolaryngol Head Neck Surg 1997;117(3):S1–7.
13. Keir J. Why do we have paranasal sinuses? J Laryngol Otol 2009;123(1):4–8.
14. Pelikan Z, Pelikan-Filipek M. Role of nasal allergy in chronic maxillary sinusitis—diagnostic value of nasal challenge with allergen. J Allergy Clin Immunol 1990;86(4):484–91.
15. Ramadan HH, Fornelli R, Ortiz AO, et al. Correlation of allergy and severity of sinus disease. Am J Rhinol 1999;13(5):345–7.

16. Osguthorpe JD. Surgical outcomes in rhinosinusitis: what we know. Otolaryngol Head Neck Surg 1999;120(4):451–3.
17. Puhakka T, Mäkelä MJ, Alanen A, et al. Sinusitis in the common cold. J Allergy Clin Immunol 1998;102(3):403–8.
18. Slack CL, Dahn KA, Abzug MJ, et al. Antibiotic-resistant bacteria in pediatric chronic sinusitis. Pediatr Infect Dis J 2001;20(3):247–50.
19. Anon JB. Acute bacterial rhinosinusitis in pediatric medicine: current issues in diagnosis and management. Pediatr Drugs 2003;5(1):25–33.
20. Hamilos DL. Chronic sinusitis. J Allergy Clin Immunol 2000;106(2):213–27.
21. Babinski D, Trawinska-Bartnicka M. Rhinosinusitis in cystic fibrosis: not a simple story. Int J Pediatr Otorhinolaryngol 2008;72(5):619–24.
22. Baroody FM. Mucociliary transport in chronic rhinosinusi- tis. Clin Allergy Immunol 2007;20:103–19.
23. Brietzke SE, Shin JJ, Choi S, et al. Clinical consensus statement: pediatric chronic rhinosinusitis. Otolaryngol Head Neck Surg 2014;151(4):542–53.
24. Leo G, Incorvaia C, Masieri S, et al. Imaging criteria for diagnosis of chronic rhinosinusitis in children. Eur Ann Allergy Clin Immunol 2010;42(6):199–204.
25. Lund VJ, Kennedy DW. Quantification for staging sinusitis. The Staging and Therapy Group. Ann Otol Rhinol Laryngol Suppl 1995;167:17–21.
26. Bhattacharyya N, Jones DT, Hill M, et al. The diagnostic accuracy of computed tomography in pediatric chronic rhinosinusitis. Arch Otolaryngol Head Neck Surg 2004;130(9):1029–32.
27. Varshney R, Lee JT, Varshney R, et al. Current trends in topical therapies for chronic rhinosinusitis: update and literature review. Expert Opin Drug Deliv 2017;14(2):257–71.
28. Harvey R, Hannan SA, Badia L, et al. Nasal saline irrigations for the symptoms of chronic rhinosinusitis. Cochrane Database Syst Rev 2007;(3):CD006394.
29. Jeffe JS, Bhushan B, Schroeder JW Jr. Nasal saline irrigation in children: a study of compliance and tolerance. Int J Pediatr Otorhinolaryngol 2012;76(3):409–13.
30. Ozturk F, Bakirtas A, Ileri F, et al. Efficacy and tolerability of systemic methylpred- nisolone in children and adolescents with chronic rhinosinusitis: a double-blind, placebo-controlled randomized trial. J Allergy Clin Immunol 2011;128(2):348–52.
31. Phipps CD, Wood WE, Gibson WS, et al. Gastroesophageal reflux contributing to chronic sinus disease in children: a prospective analysis. Arch Otolaryngol Head Neck Surg 2000;126(7):831–6.
32. Kuruvilla M, de la Morena MT, Kuruvilla M, et al. Antibiotic prophylaxis in primary immune deficiency disorders. J Allergy Clin Immunol Pract 2013;1(6):573–82.
33. Bhenke J, Jimenez-Herrera P, Peppers B, et al. Outcome of Immunoglobulin Replacement Therapy in Children with Rhinosinusitis. Int Forum Allergy Rhinol 2021. https://doi.org/10.1002/alr.22921.
34. Cornet ME, Georgalas C, Reinartz SM, et al. Long-term results of functional endo- scopic sinus surgery in children with chronic rhinosinusitis with nasal polyps. Rhi- nology 2013;51(4):328–34.
35. Vandenberg SJ, Heatley DG. Efficacy of adenoidectomy in relieving symptoms of chronic sinusitis in children. Arch Otolaryngol Head Neck Surg 1997;123(7):675–8.
36. Ramadan HH. Adenoidectomy vs endoscopic sinus surgery for the treatment of pediatric sinusitis. Arch Otolaryngol Head Neck Surg 1999;125(11):1208–11.
37. Ramadan HH. Cost JL, "Outcome of adenoidectomy versus adenoidectomy with maxillary sinus wash for chronic rhinosinusitis in children. Laryngoscope 2008; 118(5):871–3.

38. Ramadan HH, Makary C.A.. Can Computed tomography score predict outcome of adenoidectomy for chronic rhinosinusitis in children. Am J Rhinol Allergy 2014; 28(1):80–2.
39. Ramadan HH, Terrell AM. Balloon catheter sinuplasty and adenoidectomy in children with chronic rhinosinusitis. Ann Otol Rhinol Laryngol 2010;119(9):578–82.
40. Zalzal HG, Makary CA, Ramadan HH. Long-Term Effectiveness of Balloon Catheter Sinuplasty in Pediatric Chronic Maxillary Sinusitis. Ear Nose Throat J 2019; 98(4):207–11.
41. Senior BA, Kennedy DW, Tanabodee J, et al. Long-term results of functional endoscopic sinus surgery. Laryngoscope 1998;108(2):151–7.
42. Mair EA, Bolger WE, Breisch EA. Sinus and facial growth after pediatric endoscopic sinus surgery. Arch Otolaryngol Head Neck Surg 1995;121(5):547–52.
43. Bothwell MR, Piccirillo JF, Lusk RP, et al. Long-term outcome of facial growth after functional endoscopic sinus surgery. Otolaryngol Head Neck Surg 2002;126(6): 628–34.
44. Makary CA, Ramadan HH. The role of sinus surgery in children. Laryngoscope 2013;123(6):1348–52.
45. Vlastarakos PV, Fetta M, Segas JV, et al. Functional endoscopic sinus surgery improves sinus-related symptoms and quality of life in children with chronic rhinosinusitis: a systematic analysis and meta-analysis of published interventional studies. Clin Pediatr 2013;52(12):1091–7.

Nasal Obstruction in the Infant

Samantha Frank, MD[a],*, Scott R. Schoem, MD, MBA[b]

KEYWORDS

- Nasal obstruction • Neonatal rhinitis • Nasal stenosis • Congenital nasal masses

KEY POINTS

- Complete nasal obstruction includes the diagnoses of arhinia and bilateral choanal atresia. Most infant nasal obstruction is partial.
- Mirror test and passage of small 5 or 6F catheters are used to assess nasal patency. Flexible nasal endoscopy is commonly performed by otolaryngologists to determine the cause of obstruction.
- Birth trauma can lead to septal deviation, which often self-corrects.
- Nasal stenosis includes anterior stenosis (pyriform aperture stenosis), midnasal stenosis, and posterior stenosis (choanal atresia). Treatment varies from conservative steroid drops to surgical intervention.
- Congenital nasal masses require evaluation by an otolaryngologist with subsequent medical or surgical treatment based on diagnosis.

INTRODUCTION

Neonatal nasal obstruction is a common condition. Neonates have commonly been referred to in older literature as "obligate nasal breathers." However, when an infant is suffering from complete nasal obstruction, they will experience cyanosis followed by a forced opening of their mouth to breathe orally. This cycle will continue to allow for ventilation.[1–3] Therefore, the term "preferential nasal breathers" has been introduced as the more accurate term.

NASAL PHYSIOLOGY

The functions of the nose include flow of air, filtration, and olfaction.[4,5] As the air flows through the nasal cavity, it is heated and humidified. The cilia of the nose work to filter

The authors had no funding for this work. They do not have any financial or commercial interests to disclose.

[a] Department of Surgery, Division of Otolaryngology–Head & Neck Surgery, University of Connecticut, 263 Farmington Avenue, Farmington, CT 06030, USA; [b] Connecticut Children's, 282 Washington Street, Hartford, CT 06106, USA
* Corresponding author.
E-mail address: sfrank@uchc.edu

inhaled particles, including microbes. The sinuses, which vary in number based on developmental age, drain their contents through the nasal cavities. Olfaction via cranial nerve I occurs at the olfactory cleft. The nose maintains mucous flow in order to perform the functions of filtration as well as olfaction.

The nasal mucosa has a large supply of arterioles and arteriovenous anastomoses that drain into venous sinusoids. These sinusoids carry sympathetic and parasympathetic innervation. During sympathetic activation, sympathetic fibers are activated by norepinephrine to decrease blood flow via the sinusoids with resultant venous return and decreased congestion. Conversely, during parasympathetic activation, parasympathetic fibers work by acetylcholine to increase congestion. Sensory C fibers are activated via neurokinin A and substance P to downregulate sympathetic response and increase congestion.[6] Normal physiologic function is hindered when anatomic or mucosal aberrations affect the nasal cavity.[7] Even minor increases in mucovascular edema can result in significantly decreased airflow.[8]

CLINICAL EVALUATION

A complete history focusing on onset, severity, and attempted treatments is crucial. The clinician should ascertain triggers, resolving factors, as well as relieving factors.

Concerning signs, such as cyanosis, must be assessed. Cyclical cyanosis can occur in the setting of complete obstruction. This presents with a cycle of cyanosis when the neonate cannot breathe through the nose, followed by opening of the mouth for breathing via a cry, which temporarily resolves the cyanosis. In these patients, an oral airway may temporize the situation. A history of complete obstruction with cyanosis typically will lead to the diagnosis of bilateral choanal atresia. Conversely, most patients will experience varying degrees of partial obstruction.

The complete nasal examination of the neonate involves observation of breathing at rest and with feeding. The presence of stertor, which is described as a low-pitched, inspiratory noise, should be noted as well. This noise indicates turbulent airflow with vibration of nasopharyngeal and/or oropharyngeal soft tissue, which is often indicative of nasal obstruction. A mirror test can be performed to assess airflow by placing the mirror under each nostril separately. If the mirror fogs, airflow via that nostril is confirmed. A large mirror can be used to assess both nostrils simultaneously, with the expectation of 2 areas of fogging if there is patency of bilateral nasal cavities. A small 5 or 6F catheter can be passed via each nostril to ensure patency. This test should be interpreted with caution, however, as a false positive result may be concluded when the catheter prematurely makes contact with the inferior turbinate, prohibiting further passage despite nasal patency. Alternatively, a false negative result may be concluded when the catheter appears to pass when merely coiling within the nasal cavity. Flexible nasal endoscopy is commonly performed by the otolaryngologist and can ascertain presence of masses and location of obstruction. Although rigid flexible nasal endoscopy is the superior evaluation performed in adults to evaluate nasal obstruction, flexible nasal endoscopy is more feasible than rigid nasal endoscopy in the evaluation of nasal obstruction in the neonate.

Imaging may be warranted in select cases and can include computed tomography (CT) scan or MRI scan, with or without intravenous contrast. CT is more helpful in the assessment of bony abnormalities, such as pyriform aperture stenosis and choanal atresia. MRI lends superior soft tissue imaging capabilities and is useful for defining masses, and especially for determining intracranial extent. Antenatal fetal MRI has been extremely useful in identifying masses of the head and neck that may cause obstruction before birth. This imaging modality can further define those masses identified on fetal ultrasonography, assisting in surgical planning, allowing for surgical intervention shortly after birth.[9]

BIRTH TRAUMA

Birth trauma altering the structure of the nose, including external nasal deformity or significant nasal septal deviation, has been reported to occur in 1% to 2% of births.[10] However, most of these neonates will not exhibit symptoms, so this is a much less common clinical entity. Two mechanisms of action have been suggested regarding these traumas. Isolated anterior septal deviations have been purported to be the result of trauma in the birth canal. These cases are more likely to show external nasal deformity. In cases of combined anterior and posterior septal deviations, these are thought to be due to transmitted intrauterine forces during fetal skull molding. Studies have demonstrated an increased incidence of septal deformity in complicated or difficult deliveries.[11] The deviation is often minor and self-corrects within several weeks after birth. In rare cases, the septum is deviated to such a degree that normal nasal breathing is not possible. In this case, closed reduction is required in the first week after birth.

MEDICATION-INDUCED RHINITIS

Placental blood flow allows the transmission of medications and drug metabolites. Some of these may lead to nasal congestion, including several classes of antihypertensives and antidepressants, as well as illicit substances such as cocaine. Therefore, maternal medication history is an important part of the history in the evaluation of neonatal nasal obstruction. Treatment should be aimed at identifying and eliminating the causative agent.

NEONATAL RHINITIS

Neonatal rhinitis is a common newborn condition that presents with clear or mucoid rhinorrhea with nasal mucosal edema in the afebrile newborn. Neonates will demonstrate stertor, poor feeding, and respiratory distress. There will be no history or examination findings consistent with infectious or anatomic causes in these cases. It is physiologic in nature with parasympathetic response overtaking the sympathetic response. Mast cells, eosinophils, basophils, and goblet cells release local inflammatory mediators, including histamine, kinins, prostaglandins, arachidonic acid metabolites, and mucin, that contribute to rhinitis.[8]

Parents often present to clinic with newborns in the setting of neonatal rhinitis. Mucosal edema can be a result of various underlying pathologic conditions, including allergy, laryngopharyngeal reflux, infection, or a medication side effect.

The treatment is conservative in nature and includes initiation of a topical decongestant, such as oxymetazoline or neosynephrine, as well as topical nasal steroids in addition to nasal saline drops and bulb suctioning. Many of these cases will respond to this conservative management, and those that do not respond may require further evaluation for an alternate cause.[5]

CONGENITAL NASAL ABNORMALITIES
Arhinia

Congenital arhinia (or arrhinia) lends to a clear diagnosis (**Fig. 1**; **Table 1**). Prenatal diagnosis is often elucidated by abnormal facial profile on fetal ultrasonography. It is one of 2 causes of complete nasal obstruction and consists of the absence of the external nose, nasal cavities, and olfactory apparatus. It is an exceedingly rare

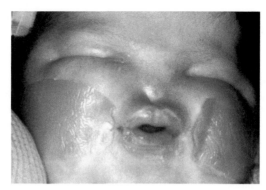

Fig. 1. Infant with arhinia. (Reprinted/adapted by permission from Springer Nature Customer Service Centre GmbH: Springer Nature Disorders of the Nasal Cavity by Scott R. Schoem 2015.)

condition and occurs as a result of failed fusion of the maxillary process and lateral nasal processes at 3 to 8 weeks of gestation. Congenital arhinia includes total arhinia, hemi-arhinia, and proboscis lateralis.[12] Hypertelorism, microphthalmia, palatal abnormalities, cryptorchidism, and blindness may be associated conditions.[13]

Neonates with arhinia will experience lack of olfaction as well, given failures of cribriform plate fusion in utero leading to olfactory agenesis. Although the congenital deformity is significant, patients will often have normal intelligence. Initial management varies based on the degree of respiratory distress. Neonates with mild symptoms may require only an oral airway and/or orogastric feeding. Those with more severe symptoms may necessitate a tracheostomy for a safe airway. Surgical correction is challenging and requires a multidisciplinary team of otolaryngology, plastic surgery, and possibly neurosurgery to establish nasal patency and perform external nasal reconstruction.[14] CT and MRI are both useful imaging studies used for surgical planning.[15]

Anterior (Pyriform Aperture) Stenosis

Congenital nasal pyriform aperture stenosis (CNPAS) is a rare diagnosis, occurring in about 1 in 25,000 births.[16] The pyriform aperture is defined as the opening between the lateral nasal process of the maxilla, the horizontal process of the maxilla, and

Table 1
Evaluation and management approaches to congenital nasal abnormalities

Diagnosis	Type of Obstruction	Evaluation	Management Approaches
Arhinia	Complete	CT MRI	Surgical intervention
Pyriform aperture stenosis	Partial	Nasal endoscopy CT	Topical steroids Surgical intervention (urethral sound dilation, sublabial drill out, possible stent placement)
Midnasal stenosis	Partial	Nasal endoscopy CT	Topical steroids Possible surgical intervention
Choanal atresia	Partial (unilateral) Complete (bilateral)	Nasal endoscopy CT	Surgical intervention likely in 2 stages

the anterior nasal spine inferiorly. It is the most anterior nasal opening of the nasal airway. CNPAS has been theorized to be due to either defective formation of the primary palate during embryogenesis or bony overgrowth of the nasal process of the maxilla.[17] Severity of anatomic defect can vary from mild to complete atresia.[18] Patients will present with stertor and difficulty coordinating breathing and feeding with mild stenosis. If stenosis is severe, it can mimic choanal atresia, as the patient may experience respiratory distress with cyclical cyanosis as well as inability to feed. On examination, the mirror test will be positive, as there remains some airflow. Often, a catheter will not pass, and nasal endoscopy cannot be performed because of the level of stenosis.

Pyriform aperture stenosis is a result of a midline deformity and can therefore be accompanied with holoprosencephaly defects, including single central incisor, absent upper labial frenulum, and absence of the corpus collosum.[19,20] This is accompanied with pituitary dysfunction with subsequent dysfunction of the hypothalamic-pituitary-adrenal axis. There is a large spectrum of presentation, and pyriform aperture stenosis can be isolated.

CT imaging should be performed and will reveal evidence of narrowing at the pyriform aperture. A normal full-term neonate will have a width of 11 mm or greater between the nasal processes of the maxilla at the level of the inferior meatus.[21] CT will also aid in ruling out other midline abnormalities (**Fig. 2**).

Treatment varies based on clinical severity. If stenosis is isolated and mild, topical steroid drops, such as 0.1% dexamethasone, may be used.[22] 1% Prednisolone acetate drops have been used as an alternative, as these are much weaker with a decreased risk of adrenal suppression. In syndromic patients, they may need airway management with tracheostomy and surgical intervention.

Conservative surgical intervention may include urethral sound dilation. If more significant surgical correction is necessary, a sublabial approach may be used to drill out

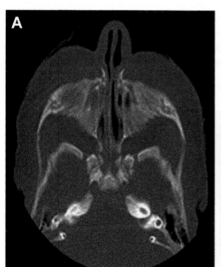
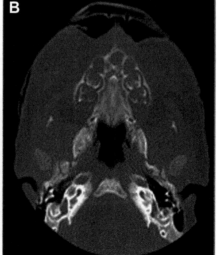

Fig. 2. CT scan of patient with pyriform aperture stenosis. (*A*) Anterior nasal obstruction apparent on CT. (*B*) Single central incisor demonstrated. (Reprinted/adapted by permission from Springer Nature Customer Service Centre GmbH: Springer Nature Disorders of the Nasal Cavity by Scott R. Schoem 2015.)

the maxillary process and widen the pyriform aperture.[23] Stents are often placed, but success has been reported without the use of stents.[24]

Midnasal Stenosis

Midnasal stenosis presents as a congenital thickening of the nasal septum or bony narrowing of the nasal cavity. The diagnosis should be confirmed with CT scan, which will demonstrate an obstruction between the mucosa of the inferior turbinate and septum.[16] It is a self-limited condition. Good effect can often be achieved with treatment of topical steroids with the possible addition of continuous positive airway pressure.[25] Treatment should include mild steroid drops with dexamethasone or prednisolone acetate drops. Severe cases have been reported necessitating surgical intervention with nasal endoscopy and dilation of the stenotic segment.[26]

Posterior (Choanal) Stenosis and Atresia

Choanal atresia occurs in 1 in 5000 to 9000 births. It results as either failure of buccopharyngeal membrane breakdown with persistence of the mesoderm or with misdirection of the mesoderm. Both male and female neonates are diagnosed with choanal atresia with equal distribution.[27,28] Atresia is unilateral in 2 of 3 of cases, with the right side more commonly involved.[16] Ninety percent of atresia is bony, and 10% is membranous only.

Bilateral choana atresia is a medical emergency. However, emergent surgical management is not required. Neonates classically present with cyclical cyanosis in which neonates are unable to breathe transnasally with subsequent crying to force mouth breathing and continuation of this cycle once the mouth closes. An oral airway can be placed to provide patency of the mouth for breathing, although this is often not tolerated in fully awake patients. Orogastric feeding can be initiated to allow for adequate nutrition. As described previously, diagnosis can be made with the assistance of a mirror or 5 or 6F catheter. Subsequent flexible fiber-optic endoscopy is often diagnostic. Fine-cut CT scan is necessary to determine the site and degree of obstruction (**Fig. 3**A). The nasopharynx should be imaged as well as rarely an obstructing nasal or nasopharyngeal mass may mimic choanal atresia. CT scan is also helpful to determine the relationship of the skull base to the nasopharynx. In certain conditions, such as Treacher Collins, the space between the posterior nasal cavity and the nasopharynx is greatly reduced by a down-sloping skull base, which leads to

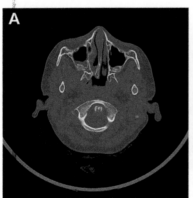
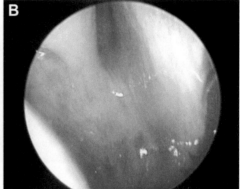

Fig. 3. Choanal atresia. (A) CT scan demonstrating unilateral right-sided choanal atresia. (B) Nasal endoscopy demonstrating complete choanal atresia.

difficulty creating a sufficient opening from the posterior nasal cavity to the naso-pharynx without restenosis. Unilateral atresia often does not present until childhood or adolescence and presents as a unilateral nasal obstruction with unilateral rhinorrhea.

Choanal atresia can occur as part of the constellation of defects in CHARGE syndrome, which includes ocular Colobomas, Heart defects, choanal Atresia, Restricted growth, Genitourinary hypoplasia, and Ear abnormalities. Heart defects occur in 75% to 85% of patients. Ear abnormalities, including ossicular malformations, cochlear anomalies, and semicircular canal hypoplasia, occur in more than 80% of patients. Patients may also demonstrate tracheoesophageal fistula.[29] This syndrome results because of an abnormality of the CHD7 marker on chromosome 8q12.2, which encodes chromodomain helicase DNA binding protein. CHD7 analysis detects mutations in 65% to 70% of affected individuals.

Surgical repair of choanal atresia varies depending on bony involvement. Trans-nasal endoscopic surgical repair is the preferred approach and is performed in stages (**Fig. 3**B). In the first-stage surgery, the posterior nasal septum/vomer is removed. Stents may be placed, but it has been preferable to avoid use of stents.[23–33] The second-stage surgery should occur 3 to 4 weeks later to remove resultant granulation tissue. Steroid-eluting stents have been trialed as an alternate method to avoid second-stage surgery.[34] If unilateral atresia is diagnosed early, surgical intervention should be delayed until at least age 6 months if possible.[35]

CONGENITAL MASSES
Infantile Hemangioma

Infantile hemangioma is the most common neoplasm of infancy (**Table 2**). They may be found anywhere throughout the body, but are most common in the head and neck, specifically within the midface. Their growth is rapid early in life with endothelial cell proliferation followed by gradual involution. With rapid proliferation, these may cause nasal obstruction and subsequent respiratory distress. Many treatment modalities had been reported, including intralesional corticosteroid injections, systemic corticosteroids, and laser ablation. However, recent research is concurrent with

Table 2		
Key findings and management approaches to congenital nasal masses		
Diagnosis	**Key Findings**	**Management Approaches**
Infantile hemangioma	Rapid early growth with subsequent involution	Beta-blocker therapy (atenolol current preference)
Nasolacrimal duct cyst	Round masses at Hasner valve or inferomedial to medial canthus	Duct probing Balloon dilation Intranasal endoscopic marsupialization with or without stent placement
Meningocele/ meningoencephalocele	Soft, compressible, pulsatile intranasal or extranasal mass	Surgical intervention with Otolaryngology and Neurosurgery
Glioma	Firm, noncompressible, nonpulsatile intranasal or extranasal mass	Surgical intervention (intranasal approach for intranasal lesions)
Nasal dermoid	Midline nasal mass, often only extranasal	Surgical intervention with possible neurosurgical assistance

hemangiomas in other locations, which consists of beta-blocker therapy. This blocks endothelial cell proliferation and migration, inhibits formation of the actin cytoskeleton, and alters vascular endothelial growth factor receptors.[36] Propranolol had been the treatment of choice, but recent research demonstrates that atenolol has similar efficacy with a more limited side-effect profile. Therefore, atenolol has become the preferred beta-blocker therapy.[37–40]

Nasolacrimal Duct Cyst (Dacryocystocele)

Nasolacrimal duct obstruction is common in the neonate.[41,42] This is often incomplete in nature and resolves spontaneously with conservative manage by 1 year of age. Nasolacrimal duct cysts are round masses visualized at Hasner valve (**Fig. 4**A). Patients will present with unilateral partial obstruction. A round mass will be seen lateral to the inferior turbinate in the anterior nasal cavity on examination.[43] Obstruction may alternatively occur proximally, which would present as a gray-blue mass inferomedially to the medial canthus. Bilateral dacryocystocele is rare, but well documented. This entity presents as a more complete nasal obstruction with respiratory distress.[44,45]

CT scan will reveal a cystic structure of the nasolacrimal duct (**Fig. 4**B). Treatment varies based on severity of presentation. Unilateral obstruction rarely requires surgical intervention, whereas bilateral obstruction may require more urgent surgical intervention. Surgical intervention may range from duct probing or balloon dilation to intranasal endoscopic marsupialization with dacryocystorhinostomy and silastic tubing placement.[46,47] Nasal endoscopy has been reported as a useful adjunct during intervention.[48] Dacryoendoscopy can be used in refractory cases.[49] The silastic stent is removed 3 to 6 weeks following surgery.

Meningocele/Meningoencephalocele

A meningocele is an anterior inferior outpouching of the meninges into the nasal cavity owing to small defects in the floor of the intracranial cavity. A meningoencephalocele is an outpouching that includes meninges as well as brain in the setting of a larger defect. This may present with an external lesion at the region of the glabella. It may alternatively be intranasal in nature with protrusion only through the cribriform plate and on examination may resemble a nasal polyp. These masses are soft, compressible, and pulsatile on examination. On examination, the mass will increase in size with compression of the jugular vein or with Valsalva maneuver or strain.

Imaging must be performed. CT will identify a bony defect within the skull base. MRI will show an intranasal mass that is isointense or hypointense with T1

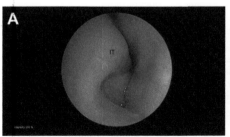 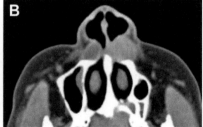

Fig. 4. Nasolacrimal duct cyst. (A) Nasal endoscopy showing right nasolacrimal duct cyst at the level of Hasner's valve; inferior turbinate (IT). (B) CT scan demonstrating bilateral nasolacrimal duct cysts.

sequence and hyperintense with T2 sequence. MRI will help to determine possible intracranial extension. Surgical intervention requires a combined approach with otolaryngology and neurosurgery, and surgery is usually performed via anterior frontal craniotomy.[50]

Glioma

A glioma represents a mass of heterotopic glial tissue. This tissue is intermixed with fibrous and vascular connective tissue that gives a firm structure to the lesion. In 10% to 15% of cases, there is a fibrous stalk extending to the skull base, but these will only very rarely have a patent meningeal connection. Patients present with a unilateral nasal obstruction. These can be noted within the nasal cavity or the nasopharynx (**Fig. 5**). Sixty percent is extranasal; 30% is intranasal, and 10% is combined with a dumbbell growth pattern. It is a firm, noncompressible, and nonpulsatile mass, which is well differentiated from meningocele or meningoencephalocele. As with meningocele or meningoencephalocele, CT scan and MR imaging are helpful to determine the site of the lesion and intracranial extent. Surgery is the mainstay of treatment and is performed via an intranasal approach for intranasal lesions.[51,52] Neurosurgery is often not required given its exclusive intranasal approach but should be easily available for any unexpected complication.

Nasal Dermoid

Nasal dermoid cysts or sinuses are derived from ectodermal and mesodermal tissue that forms as a remnant in the prenasal space posterior to the nasal bones and anterior to the nasal and septal cartilages. The sinus tract is identified with a pit and may be related with a hair tuft on the nasal dorsum. There may be associated infection or keratin discharge. A nasal dermoid is a midline abnormality that is usually accompanied with outward physical deformity. There is usually no obstruction.

CT scan can define bony defects in the skull base and can reveal widening of the crista galli that is indicative of potential intracranial extension. MRI is a useful adjunct to determine extent of the lesion, including intracranial extent (**Fig. 6**).[53] Imaging will identify presence of a tract in the case of a dermal sinus. If no intracranial extent is identified, surgical intervention may be accomplished via nasal approach with neurosurgical assistance nearby. This may be achieved via endoscopic closed approach, external rhinoplasty, or open approach.[54–56] If intracranial extent has been identified,

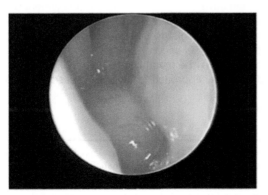

Fig. 5. Endoscopic view of nasopharyngeal glioma. (Reprinted/adapted by permission from Springer Nature Customer Service Centre GmbH: Springer Nature Disorders of the Nasal Cavity by Scott R. Schoem 2015.)

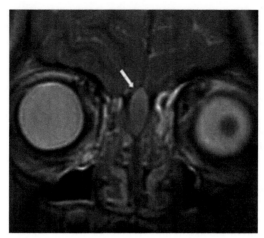

Fig. 6. MRI scan demonstrating nasal dermoid (arrow) with borders revealing lack of intracranial extent.

an endoscopic transnasal approach may still be appropriate, but neurosurgical assistance is recommended in case of unexpected complications.[57]

Other Tumors

Rarely, tumors identified within the nasal cavity or nasopharynx may be unrecognized. This can be in the setting of benign or malignant teratoma, hairy polyp, or other fibrous tissue tumors.[58–61] These tumors can occur anywhere within the nasal cavity. They are often identified on fetal ultrasound. Polyhydramnios may be present because of impaired fetal swallowing. Fetal MRI is necessary to determine the site and degree of obstruction to plan for management.

FETAL NASAL OBSTRUCTION

In cases of identified obstruction on fetal ultrasound and/or fetal MRI, a safe approach must be planned. This may necessitate urgent surgical intervention for airway management. The ex utero intrapartum treatment approach is a multidisciplinary approach that facilitates safe, effective, and prompt airway management with or without tumor excision after delivery.[62] This approach is a combined effort between neonatology, obstetrics, and an otolaryngologist to use maternal-fetal circulation as maintenance oxygenation while an airway is secured in the neonate. Reports demonstrate that maternal-fetal circulation may be maintained for up to 1 hour. This approach can be a lifesaving multidisciplinary approach to obstructive lesions discovered in utero.[63]

CLINICS CARE POINTS

- Most nasal obstruction is partial. Cyclical cyanosis seen with complete obstruction is typically, but not exclusively, seen in cases of bilateral choanal atresia.
- Causes of partial obstruction include neonatal rhinitis, trauma-induced structural abnormalities, congenital structural abnormalities, and congenital masses.
- In the pediatric clinic, a mirror fog test or passage of a small catheter via the nasal cavities can inform patency. However, be aware of false positives and negatives.

- Imaging can be helpful. Computed tomography imaging can define bony abnormalities in disorders, such as pyriform aperture stenosis and choanal atresia. MRI provides better soft tissue definition and is useful for defining masses.
- Neonatal rhinitis and mild stenosis can be treated conservatively with topical nasal decongestants and topical nasal steroids.
- Infantile hemangioma is treated with beta-blocker therapy.
- Arhinia, more significant nasal stenosis, choanal atresia, and the presence of congenital masses other than infantile hemangioma will require surgical intervention.
- Fetal ultrasound and fetal MRI can be used to detect obstructive lesions before birth. A subsequent ex utero intrapartum treatment procedure can be planned by a multidisciplinary team.

REFERENCES

1. Bergeson PS, Shaw JC. Are infants really obligate nasal breathers? Clin Pediatr 2001;40:567–9.
2. Miller M, Martin R, Carlo W, et al. Oral breathing in newborn infants. J Pediatr 1985;107:465–9.
3. Trabalon M, Schaal B. It takes a mouth to eat and a nose to breathe: abnormal oral respiration affects neonates' oral competence and systemic adaptation. Int J Pediatr 2012;2012:207605.
4. Leong S, Chen X, Lee H, et al. A review of the implications of computational fluid dynamic studies on nasal airflow and physiology. Rhinology 2010;48:139–45.
5. Nathan C, Seid A. Neonatal rhinitis. Int J Pediatr Otorhinolaryngol 1997;14:59–65.
6. Anggard A, Edwall L. The effects of sympathetic nerve stimulation on the tracer disappearance rate and local blood content in the nasal mucosa of the cat. Acta Otolaryngol 1974;77:131–9.
7. Wang D, Lee H, Gordon B. Impacts of fluid dynamics simulations in study of nasal airflow physiology and pathophysiology in realistic human three-dimensional nose models. Clin Exp Otorhinolaryngol 2012;5:181–7.
8. Davis SS, Eccles R. Nasal congestion: mechanisms, measurement and medications. Core information for the clinician. Clin Otolaryngol 2004;29:659–66.
9. Grzegorczyk V, Brasseur-Daudruy M, Labadie G, et al. Prenatal diagnosis of a nasal glioma. Pediatr Radiol 2010;40(10):1706–9.
10. Metzenbaum M. "Dislocation of the lower end of the nasal septal cartilage: a treatise dealing with dislocations of the lower end of the nasal septal cartilage in the new-born (injury sustained at birth), in infants and in young children and with their anatomic replacement by orthopedic procedures," Archives of Otolaryngology. Head Neck Surg 1936;24(1):78–88.
11. Emami AJ, Brodsky L, Pizzuto M. Neonatal septoplasty: case report and review of the literature. Int J Pediatr Otorhinolaryngol 1996;35(3):271–5.
12. Tessier P, Ciminello F, Wolfe S. The arrhinias. Scand J Plast Reconstr Surg 2009; 43:177–96.
13. Graham J, Lee J. Bosma arhinia microphthalmia syndrome. Am J Med Genet 2006;140:189–93.
14. Fuller AK, McCrary HC, Graham ME, et al. The case of the missing nose: congenital arrhinia case presentation and management recommendations. Ann Otol Rhinol Laryngol 2020;129(7):645–8.
15. Goyal A, Agrawal V, Raina VK, et al. Congenital arhinia: a rare case. J Indian Assoc Pediatr Surg 2008;13(4):153–4.

16. Galluzzi F, Garavello W, Dalfino G, et al. Congenital bony nasal cavity stenosis: a review of current trends in diagnosis and treatment. Int J Pediatr Otorhinolaryngol 2021;144:110670.

17. Rao A, Godehal SM, Patil AR, et al. Congenital nasal pyriform aperture stenosis: a rare cause of neonatal nasal airway obstruction. BJR Case Rep 2015;1(1). https://dpoi.org/20150006.

18. Angulo C, Jayawardena ADL, Caruso PA, et al. Congenital nasal piriform aperture atresia: a case report and novel finding. Int J Pediatr Otorhinolaryngol 2020;135:110124.

19. Hui Y, Friedberg J, Crysdale W. Congenital nasal pyriform aperture stenosis as a presenting feature of holoprosencephaly. Int J Pediatr Otorhinolaryngol 1995;31:263–74.

20. Tavin E, Stecker E, Marion R. Nasal pyriform aperture stenosis and the holoprosencephaly spectrum. Int J Pediatr Otorhinolaryngol 1994;28:199–204.

21. Belden C, Mancuso A, Schmalfuss I. CT features of congenital nasal piriform aperture stenosis: initial experience. Radiology 1999;213:495–501.

22. Collins B, Powitzky R, Enix J, et al. Congenital nasal pyriform aperture stenosis: conservative management. Ann Otol Rhinol Laryngol 2013;122(10):601–4.

23. Merea VS, Lee AHY, Peron DL, et al. CPAS: surgical approach with combined sublabial bone resection and inferior turbinate reduction without stents. Laryngoscope 2015;125(6):1460–4.

24. Wine TM, Dedhia K, Chi DH. Congenital nasal pyriform aperture stenosis: is there a role for nasal dilation? JAMA Otolaryngol Head Neck Surg 2014;140(4):352–6.

25. Onder SS, Sahin-Yilmaz A, Tinay OG, et al. Congenital midnasal stenosis: conservative management. Int J Pediatr Otorhinolaryngol 2020;132:109939.

26. Raghavan U, Fuad F, Gibbin KP. Congenital midnasal stenosis in an infant. Int J Pediatr Otorhinolaryngol 2004;68:823–5.

27. Harris J, Robert E, Kallen B. Epidemiology of choanal atresia with special reference to the CHARGE association. Pediatrics 1997;99:363–7.

28. Hengerer A, Brickman T, Jeyakumar A. Choanal atresia: embryologic analysis and evolution of treatment, a 30-year experience. Laryngoscope 2008;118:862–6.

29. Bauer P, Wippold F, Goldin J, et al. Cochlear implantation in children with CHARGE association. Arch Otolaryngol Head Neck Surg 2002;128:1013–7.

30. Schoem S. Transnasal endoscopic repair of choanal atresia: why stent? Otolaryngol Head Neck Surg 2004;131:362–6.

31. El-Ahl M, El-Anwar M. Stentless endoscopic transnasal repair of bilateral choanal atresia starting with resection of vomer. Int J Pediatr Otorhinolaryngol 2012;76:1002–6.

32. De Freitas R, Berkowitz R. Bilateral choanal atresia repair in neonates – a single surgeon experience. Int J Pediatr Otorhinolaryngol 2012;76:873–8.

33. Bedwell J, Choi S. Are stents necessary after choanal atresia repair? Laryngoscope 2012;122:2365–6.

34. Wilcox LJ, Smith MM, de Alarcon A, et al. Use of steroid-eluting stents after endoscopic repair of choanal atresia: a case series with review. Ann Otol Rhinol Laryngol 2020;129(10):1003–10.

35. Moreddu E, Rizzi M, Adil E, et al. International pediatric otolaryngology group (IPOG) consensus recommendations: diagnosis, pre-operative, operative, and post-operative pediatric choanal atresia care 2019;123:151–5.

36. Stiles J, Amaya C, Pham R, et al. Propranolol treatment of infantile hemangioma endothelial cells: a molecular analysis. Exp Ther Med 2012;4:594–604.

37. Leaute-Labreze C, Dumas de la Roque E, Hubiche T, et al. Propranolol for severe hemangiomas of infancy. N Engl J Med 2008;12:2649–51.

38. Sans V, Dumas de la Roque E, Berge J, et al. Propranolol for severe infantile hemangiomas: follow up report. Pediatrics 2009;124:e423–31.

39. Parikh S, Darrow D, Grimmer J, et al. Propranolol use for infantile hemangiomas: American Society of Pediatric Otolaryngology vascular anomalies task force practice patterns. JAMA Otolaryngol Head Neck Surg 2013;139:153–6.

40. Ji Y, Chen S, Yang K, et al. Efficacy and safety of propranolol vs atenolol in infants with problematic infantile hemangiomas: a randomized clinical trial. JAMA Otolaryngol Head Neck Surg 2021;147(7):599–607.

41. Cunningham M, Woog J. Endonasal endoscopic dacryocystorhinostomy in children. Arch Otolaryngol Head Neck Surg 1998;124:328–33.

42. Guery D, Kendig E. Congenital impotency of the nasolacrimal duct. Arch Ophthalmol 1979;97:1656–8.

43. Shashy R, Durairaj V, Holmes J, et al. Congenital dacryocystocele associated with intranasal cysts: diagnosis and management. Laryngoscope 2003;113:37–40.

44. Leonard D, O'Keefe M, Rowley H, et al. Neonatal respiratory distress secondary to bilateral intranasal dacryocystoceles. Int J Pediatr Otorhinolaryngol 2008;72:1873–7.

45. Lecavalier M, Nguyen LH. Bilateral dacryocystoceles as a rare cause of neonatal respiratory distress: report of 2 cases. Ear Nose Throat J 2014;93(1):E26–8.

46. Paoli C, François M, Triglia JM, et al. Nasal obstruction in the neonate secondary to nasolacrimal duct cysts. Laryngoscope 1995;105(1):86–9.

47. Akpolat C, Sendul SY, Unal ET, et al. Outcomes of lacrimal probing surgery as the first option in the treatment of congenital dacryocystocele. Ther Adv Ophthalmol 2021;13. 25158414211030427.

48. Trott S, Colgrove N, Westgate P, et al. Systematic review of endoscopic-assisted surgical management for congenital nasolacrimal duct obstruction. Int J Pediatr Otorhinolaryngol 2020;139:110448.

49. Gupta N, Singla P, Kumar S, et al. Role of dacryoendoscopy in refractory cases of congenital nasolacrimal duct obstruction. Orbit 2020;39(3):183–9.

50. Mahapatra A, Agrawal D. Anterior encephaloceles: a series of 103 cases over 32 years. J Clin Neurosci 2006;13:536–9.

51. Rahbar R, Resto A, Robson C, et al. Nasal glioma and encephalocele: diagnosis and management. Laryngoscope 2003;113:2069–77.

52. Yokoyama M, Inouye N, Mizuno F. Endoscopic management of nasal glioma in infancy. Int J Pediatr Otorhinolaryngol 1999;51:51–4.

53. Herrington H, Adil E, Mortiz E, et al. Update on current evaluation and management of pediatric nasal dermoid. Laryngoscopy 2016;126:2151–60.

54. Holzmann D, Huisman T, Holzmann P, et al. Surgical approaches for nasal dermal sinus cysts. Rhinology 2007;45:31–5.

55. Locke R, Kubba H. The external rhinoplasty approach for congenital nasal lesions in children. Int J Pediatr Otorhinolaryngol 2011;75:337–41.

56. Winterton R, Wilks D, Chumas P, et al. Surgical correction of midline nasal dermoid sinus cysts. J Craniofac Surg 2010;21:295–300.

57. Re M, Tarchini P, Macri G, et al. Endonasal approach for intracranial nasal dermoid sinus cysts in children. Int J Pediatr Otorhinolaryngol 2012;76:1217–22.

58. Freni F, Nicastro V, Costanzo D, et al. Nasopharynx hairy polyp as a cause of stridor in newborn. J Craniofac Surg 2020;31(6):e572–4.

59. Klein A, Schoem S, Altman A, et al. Inflammatory myoblastic tumor in the neonate: a case report. Otolaryngol Head Neck Surg 2003;128:145–7.

60. Katona G, Hirschberg J, Hosszu Z, et al. Epipharyngeal teratoma in infancy. Int J Pediatr Otorhinolaryngol 1992;24:171–5.

61. Hansen J, Soerensen F, Christensen M. A five-week-old girl with inspiratory stridor due to infantile hemangiopericytoma. Eur Arch Otorhinolaryngol 2006;263: 524–7.

62. Hirose S, Farmer D, Lee H, et al. The ex utero intrapartum treatment procedure: looking back at the EXIT. J Pediatr Surg 2004;39:375–80.

63. Osborn A, Baud D, Macarthur A, et al. Multidisciplinary perinatal management of the compromised airway on placental support: lessons learned. Prenatal Diagn 2013;18:1–8.

Stridor in the Infant Patient

Habib G. Zalzal, MD[a],*, George H. Zalzal, MD[a]

KEYWORDS

- Stridor • Laryngomalacia • Supraglottoplasty • Pediatric airway
- Congenital laryngomalacia

KEY POINTS

- Stridor is defined by the harsh respiratory noise that develops owing to turbulent airflow through a restricted passage.
- Several conditions cause stridor, but laryngomalacia is the most common cause of inspiratory stridor in neonates and infants.
- Treatment of laryngomalacia depends on severity of symptoms, but most patients can be observed and will not need surgical intervention.
- Surgical treatment of severe laryngomalacia involves removal and release of collapsing supraglottic tissue with excellent results.

Video content accompanies this article at http://www.pediatric.theclinics.com.

INTRODUCTION

Stridor is a harsh respiratory noise caused by turbulent airflow through a restricted passage. At baseline, stridor is a pathologic clinical sign that should prompt a thorough investigation by the physician. Inspiratory stridor results from upper-airway obstruction resulting in prolonged inspiration in a minority of patients. Expiratory stridor, by contrast, results from lower-airway obstruction with patients exhibiting prolonged expiration. Biphasic stridor is a combination of both inspiratory and expiratory respiratory noise and typically corresponds to an obstruction in the midtracheal anatomy between the upper and lower airways. Depending on the severity of the stridor, patients may show signs of respiratory distress, including dyspnea, nasal flaring, intercostal or subcostal retractions, grunting, cyanosis, somnolence, periods of apnea, and brief resolved unexplained events (BRUEs, formerly known as acute life-threatening events or ALTEs).

The authors deny any conflict of interests or funding sources associated with this article.
[a] Division of Otolaryngology, Children's National Medical Center, 111 Michigan Avenue, Northwest, Washington, DC 20010, USA
* Corresponding author.
E-mail address: hzalzal@cnmc.org

Stridor is not a diagnosis, but a sign of a condition that can range from benign, self-limited disorders to rapidly progressing airway obstruction. Any child presenting with stridor as an acute, chronic, or recurring problem should be evaluated in a systematic and orderly manner with appropriate studies, in either an inpatient or an outpatient setting.

This article delves into the diagnosis and management of stridor in infants, with a focus on conditions resulting in inspiratory stridor secondary to laryngeal pathologic condition with an emphasis on laryngomalacia.

CAUSE AND PATHOPHYSIOLOGY

Before discussing the cause of stridor, discussion of respiratory noises of infancy must first be described, as follows:

Inspiratory stridor: High-pitched respiratory noise caused by turbulent airflow during inspiration, usually secondary to a restricted larynx or upper trachea.

Expiratory stridor: A harsh respiratory noise caused by turbulent airflow during expiration, with obstruction being within the lower airway, such as the lower trachea or bronchi.

Biphasic stridor: A harsh respiratory noise throughout the entire respiratory cycle, signaling a lesion of the midtrachea, glottis, and subglottis.

Stertor: A low-pitched, "snoring-like" respiratory noise during inspiration, typically originating from the nasopharynx.

Wheezing: A whistling respiratory noise with expiration, best heard within the lungs secondary to restricted airflow through the bronchioles.

The upper airway in children is funnel shaped, with the cricoid being the narrowest portion of the infant airway. At birth, the infant larynx is more anterior and superiorly situated than that of an adult. With growth, the larynx begins to descend, resulting in vertical elongation of the pharynx and enlargement of the upper airway. The vocal cords are approximately 6 to 8 mm long in newborns, with the subglottis having a diameter between 5 and 7 mm. The trachea itself is 4 cm long and roughly 5 mm in diameter. Once the child reaches elementary school age, the vocal cords become the narrowest segment as opposed to the cricoid and remain that way into adulthood. By adulthood, the trachea is 11 to 13 cm in length and 12 to 23 mm in width.[1]

Stridor develops via 3 air-fluid dynamic principles: Poiseuille law, Venturi effect, and Bernoulli principle. According to Poiseuille law, a 50% decrease in the radius of a tube results in an increase in flow resistance by 16 times, which produces a notable decrease in flow. With this change, the velocity of flow increases, known as the Venturi effect. The Bernoulli principle establishes that when flow velocity increases, the pressure exerted by the flow decreases, resulting in the collapse of the airway. Stridor is produced by the distortions of this laminar flow and turbulence within the reduced segment of airway anatomy, resulting in the vibratory effect of tissue.[2] For example, in laryngomalacia, inspiration of air by the child produces a negative pressure of the supraglottic tissue of the larynx, resulting in further collapse and causing pathologic stridor.[3]

DIAGNOSTIC WORKUP OF STRIDOR
History

Careful attention regarding the duration and onset of the stridor is important, especially to differentiate a chronic symptom from an acute presentation of respiratory noise, especially if there are concomitant symptoms, such as retractions or lethargy.

Chronic stridor suggests a congenital cause, such as laryngomalacia, vocal cord paresis, subglottic stenosis, vascular ring, or glottic web. Questions regarding prenatal and obstetric history are also important, as history of intubation could lead to a diagnosis of acquired subglottic stenosis if symptoms have been present for some time. If symptoms developed acutely without previous history of symptoms, foreign body aspiration is another possible cause of acute stridor. With foreign body aspiration specifically, history and physical examination are extremely important for an accurate diagnosis, as radiographic evaluation can routinely come back negative in the acute aspiration period, depending on the type of object aspirated.

Quality of the noise is also an important characteristic, as this will aid in determining the possible location of the obstruction. Time of onset of stridor is also important. Some conditions, such as subglottic hemangiomas, do not cause stridor at birth. The presence of associated symptoms is also important, particularly if the patient has a fever or cough. These can point to more infectious causes, such as laryngotracheitis, or, rarely, epiglottitis. General medical history is also important to gather, particularly if there is concern for genetic, neurologic, or craniofacial abnormalities. Stridor that worsens with crying is concerning for obstruction secondary to laryngomalacia, bilateral vocal cord paresis, subglottic stenosis, or subglottic mass, such as hemangioma. Symptoms suggestive of aspiration or coughing with feeds may indicate a laryngeal cleft. Positioning is also important to ask about, as stridor that improves with neck extension is concerning for laryngomalacia.[3]

Physical Examination and Follow-up Studies

Once a thorough history is complete, the next step in the diagnostic algorithm is physical examination (**Fig. 1**). The first part of the examination is to listen for the stridor regarding its quality, timing, positioning, and severity. Laryngeal- or trachea-based stridor is best heard with auscultation of the anterior neck. The physician must also perform a routine head and neck examination in stridulous patients. Specific attention to the nasal passages for obstruction or persistent drainage, neck musculature for enlarged lymph nodes or masses, intraoral cavity and pharynx, and a cutaneous

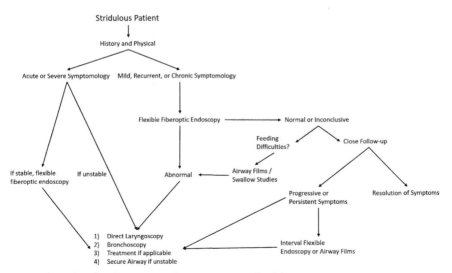

Fig. 1. Algorithm for diagnosis and management of stridor.

examination for vascular lesions are the primary areas of concern. Breathing of the child should also be noted by the physician in the event of chest retractions (intercostal, sternal, suprasternal, supraclavicular, and subxiphoid), accessory muscle use, flaring of nasal alae, neck hyperextension, and asymmetric chest motion.

Integral to evaluating the stridulous patient is the laryngeal examination. Flexible fiber-optic endoscopy to evaluate the nasopharynx and larynx has been invaluable for dynamic functional assessment of the airway in addition to rule out anatomic obstruction. The study is performed in the awake child or infant held in an upright position, typically by experienced nursing staff to prevent complications of the procedure. Topical lidocaine gel is used on all patients to reduce discomfort and pain. Nasal decongestant with topical anesthesia, such as oxymetazoline with lidocaine solution, can be applied if the nasal cavity is narrow, not allowing scope insertion, and a determination needs to be made if the reason is bony nasal stenosis or just inflammation impeding scope access. The fiber-optic endoscope can be attached to a video camera to record the procedure if necessary. The endoscope is then inserted through each side of the nose to assess nasal and choanal patency. Once cleared, the nasopharynx is examined to determine obstruction by the adenoid or congenital abnormality. The pharynx is inspected next, looking specifically at tonsillar obstruction or pooling of secretions. The supraglottic larynx is then evaluated alongside the hypopharynx, specifically evaluating for obstruction along the base of tongue, vallecula, and epiglottis. Dynamic assessment of the supraglottic larynx and the glottic larynx, in association with any stridulous noise, will help in assessing the motion and probable cause of noisy breathing should the larynx be the source. Occasionally, the subglottis and proximal trachea can be evaluated from a supraglottic view.

Radiographic studies may be performed to complement clinical examination. Plain film imaging of the anteroposterior and lateral neck are helpful in ruling out but not accurate in showing subglottic narrowing. Modified barium swallow studies are indicated in patients who have aspiration and concern for laryngeal cleft. During the initial workup for stridor, computed tomography (CT) and MRI scans are not first-line studies unless suspicion of a specific pathologic condition is highly suspected.

Operative Assessment

Definitive evaluation of the stridulous patient is the operative assessment under general anesthesia with direct laryngoscopy and bronchoscopy (**Table 1**). Both dynamic and static examination can be performed in the operative suite. Once under light anesthesia, examination of the supraglottic larynx and vocal cords can take place with

Table 1
Ancillary tests during the workup of specific causes of stridor

	Neck Airway Films	Airway Fluoroscopy	Barium Swallow	Flexible Endoscopy	Direct Laryngoscopy with Bronchoscopy
Laryngomalacia	−	−	−	++	++
Tracheomalacia	−	+	−	−	++
Subglottic stenosis	+	+	−	−	++
Vascular ring	−	−	++	−	++
Laryngeal web	−	−	−	++	++
Laryngeal cleft	−	−	+	+	++
Subglottic hemangioma	+	+	−	−	++

direct laryngoscopy. Assessment of the severity of laryngomalacia and vocal cord motion is done at this time as well, particularly if the vocal cords could not be seen on flexible endoscopy because of an obstructed view. Topical anesthesia is applied, and the rest of the airway is examined with a rigid telescope. Muscle relaxant and respiratory depressant should be avoided.[4] Thorough assessment of the hypopharynx, larynx, and tracheobronchial anatomy is performed. Instrumentation to probe the larynx may help identify laryngeal clefts and cricoarytenoid joint fixation. Video and photographic documentation of the procedure is mandatory for further review, future patient care, and risk management.

LARYNGOMALACIA IN CHILDREN

Laryngomalacia is the most common cause of stridor in neonates and infants.[5–7] Most cases follow a relatively benign course, and most patients are managed conservatively until symptoms subside by 12 to 24 months. The incidence of severe laryngomalacia resulting in persistent stridor with failure to thrive symptoms is about 10% to 15%, prompting surgical management.[5]

Pathophysiology

First described by Barthez and Rilliet[8] in 1853, 3 basic abnormalities of the larynx may be present in laryngomalacia (**Fig. 2**):

1. Elongated epiglottis that prolapses posteriorly with inspiration
2. Short aryepiglottic folds
3. Redundant supraarytenoid mucosa that prolapses anteriorly

Belmont and Grundfast[9] investigated the neurologic cause of laryngomalacia in 1984, and since then, many others have looked into the condition, but no single cause has been determined. Reflux has also been posited as a potential causative factor of laryngomalacia, as glottic edema may result in supraglottic prolapse. Persistent inflammation may result in injury to mucosal and submucosal nerves, leading to diminished laryngeal sensation and tone.[10]

Clinical Presentation

Patients with laryngomalacia will present with inspiratory stridor that intensifies with feeding, agitation, and supine positioning. Stridor may subside when the patient is

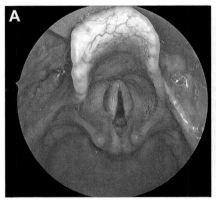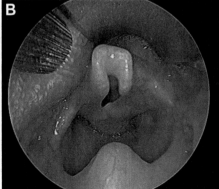

Fig. 2. Normal-appearing laryngeal anatomy (*A*) versus the appearance commonly seen in laryngomalacia (*B*).

in neck extension or when placed prone. Symptoms typically begin at birth, with an average age of presentation of around 2 weeks, but it is not uncommon for symptoms to develop later in the neonatal period.[5,11]

Airway obstruction presenting as stridor, apnea, chest/abdominal retractions, and/ or BRUEs is the most obvious constellation of symptoms for severe disease. Issues related to feeding and weight gain are the second most common indication for surgery.[12] Feeding difficulty, such as slow feeding, regurgitation, choking, or spitting up with feeds, in the setting of poor weight gain and inspiratory stridor should clue the physician to an underlying laryngeal disorder. Obstructive sleep apnea and gastroesophageal reflux disorder are commonly associated conditions with laryngomalacia that may require further evaluation. Synchronous lesions may also exist in patients with laryngomalacia and lead to multilevel obstruction. Report in the literature varies widely on the prevalence of synchronous lesions, but patients with severe laryngomalacia are more likely to have these findings than patients with milder disease.[5,13–15]

Diagnostic Testing

Flexible fiber-optic endoscopy should be the first examination performed in these patients, with the child awake and positioned upright to have an adequate visualization of the entire supraglottis and glottis. This can be performed safely in the office. Severity of the obstruction is graded by visualization of the vocal cords, where complete inability to visualize the vocal cords because of laryngeal inlet collapse of the epiglottis is a clear indication for supraglottoplasty.[16] If less than half of the vocal cords are seen, this is moderate laryngomalacia, and surgery is left to physician discretion. If more than 50% of the vocal cords are seen on flexible endoscopy, supraglottoplasty should not be performed.[16] If no laryngomalacia is identified, or if mild disease seen on flexible endoscopy does not correspond to clinical symptoms, a synchronous lesion cannot be ruled out, and direct laryngoscopy with bronchoscopy will be needed. The incidence of a synchronous lesion is around 15%, but only 5% have a significant second lesion on bronchoscopy.[13–15] Radiologic studies, such as airway fluoroscopy, have limited diagnostic utility owing to poor sensitivity.[17]

DIFFERENTIAL DIAGNOSIS OF STRIDOR

The differential for noisy breathing is wide ranging and varied depending on both age of the patient and location of the obstruction (**Table 2**; see **Fig. 2**).

Tumors and Cysts

Masses within the airway may also present with stridor. Subglottic hemangiomas are one such rare anomaly, typically found in infancy and mostly along the left side of the subglottic airway (**Fig. 3**). They are absent at birth but develop to peak size at 4 to 6 months.[1] Cutaneous lesions along the anterior neck or "beard distribution" should raise suspicion of airway hemangioma development in children who have not yet presented with airway symptoms.[18] Stridor in these patients is biphasic owing to location of the hemangioma and worsens with crying or straining as the vascular lesion becomes engorged. Historically, airway hemangiomas were treated with steroids and laser excision following diagnostic laryngoscopy and bronchoscopy.[19] Propranolol is now the mainstay of therapy for these lesions because of effectiveness and safety profile, but in recalcitrant lesions, operative intervention may still be necessary.[20] After the first year of life, most subglottic hemangiomas undergo spontaneous involution.

Supraglottic cysts, such as vallecular cysts, are congenital thin-walled mucous retention cysts that arise from the supraglottic larynx on the lingual epiglottis

Table 2
Differential diagnosis of airway obstruction based on location and age of the child

	Birth to 1 year old	1–3 years old	3–6 years old
Nasopharynx and pharynx	• Choanal atresia/stenosis • Craniofacial abnormalities • Piriform aperture stenosis • Nasal stenosis • Neonatal rhinitis	• Adenotonsillar hypertrophy • Allergic rhinitis • Foreign body	• Adenotonsillar hypertrophy • Adenoiditis • Allergic rhinitis • Foreign body
Larynx	• Laryngomalacia • Congenital cysts • Laryngeal webs • Vocal cord palsy • Subglottic stenosis (congenital & acquired) • Laryngeal cleft • Subglottic hemangioma • Reflux laryngitis	• Foreign body • Recurrent respiratory papillomatosis	• Recurrent respiratory papillomatosis • Foreign body • Epiglottitis
Trachea	• Tracheomalacia • Tracheal stenosis • Vascular compression	• Croup • Bronchiolitis • Foreign body	• Foreign body

(**Fig. 4**). Saccular cysts are similar to mucous retention cysts but can arise anteriorly to protrude within the laryngeal ventricle or laterally to extend into the false vocal cord and aryepiglottic folds. Symptoms of both conditions are dependent on size of the supraglottic cyst, which corresponds to respiratory distress severity. Subglottic cysts can mimic the stridulous presentation of subglottic hemangioma or subglottic stenosis.[21] Intubation or manipulation of the larynx is thought to be the most common cause, with 1 study finding 100% of patients who had this condition had been intubated during the neonatal period.[22] When symptomatic, treatment of this condition with marsupialization is typically performed with electrocautery, microdebrider, laser, or other microlaryngeal instrumentation. Recurrence is common, and these patients should be monitored for a period until symptoms subside.

Recurrent respiratory papillomatosis (RRP) develops in infancy and childhood in patients exposed to human papillomavirus (HPV) type 6 and 11 at birth (**Fig. 5**). This is the most common laryngeal neoplasm in children resulting in stridor. Despite early exposure, papillomas typically develop between the ages of 2 and 4 years old but can

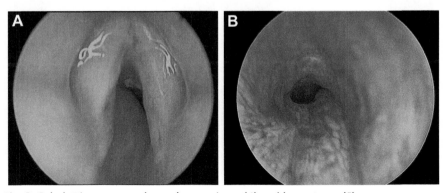

Fig. 3. Subglottic masses, such as a hemangioma (*A*) and hamartoma (*B*).

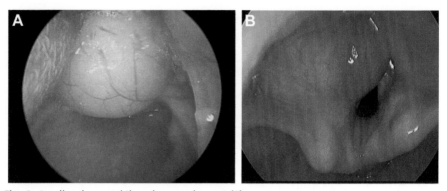

Fig. 4. A vallecular cyst (*A*) and a saccular cyst (*B*).

appear in children less than 1 year of age. Symptoms depend on the extent of the disease. Presenting symptoms are hoarseness and stridor. Treatment is with laser or microdebridement. There is no curative treatment other than periodic surgical removal. There is significant promise using the antiangiogenic agent bevacizumab for adjuvant treatment of papillomatosis, with both local injection and systemic use.[23,24] In addition, with the 2006 approval of the quadrivalent HPV vaccine, a 2018 study out of Australia found decreasing incidence of RRP in children born to vaccinated mothers over a 5-year period.[25] With the 2014 approval of the 9-valent HPV vaccine, which adds 5 more viral-like particles to the vaccine containing HPV 6, 11, 16, and 18, evidence remains to be seen if the new formulation will also lead to improved incidence rates of RRP.[26]

Vocal Cord Paralysis

The second most common cause of stridor in neonates is vocal cord paralysis.[19,27] Unilateral vocal cord paralysis and bilateral vocal cord paralysis can both present as stridor at birth, but typically bilateral vocal cord paralysis presents with much more severe respiratory distress. Unilateral vocal cord paralysis typically occurs more commonly on the left side because of the longer course of the recurrent laryngeal nerve around the aortic arch, making it more prone to iatrogenic injury and congenital cardiovascular anomalies.[28] Awake fiber-optic endoscopy of the child will allow for

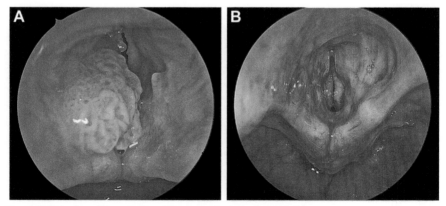

Fig. 5. RRP before (*A*) and after (*B*) removal with microdebridement.

diagnosis of this condition, but a rigid endoscopic examination also assists to rule out a pseudoparalysis, which can occur owing to vocal fold fixation rather than neurologic injury.[19] Unilateral dysfunction can be secondary to birth trauma, iatrogenic injury secondary to thoracic surgery, or masses of cardiac, pulmonary, esophageal, thyroid, or lymphoid origin. Bilateral paralysis is more likely secondary to central nervous conditions, such as Arnold-Chiari malformation, perinatal asphyxia, hydrocephalus, or cerebral hemorrhage.[28]

Workup of idiopathic vocal cord paralysis should include a CT scan or MRI scan following a course of the vagus nerve from brain to chest to rule out any lesions or abnormalities resulting in nerve compression. If no anatomic abnormality is seen, and the patient does not have a previous history of trauma or cardiovascular anomaly, a laryngeal electromyography can be performed to rule out electrical silence, but this is not necessary in neonates.[4] Approximately 73% of unilateral and 63% of bilateral vocal fold paralysis will resolve spontaneously within the first few months of life.[29,30] Recovery is typically complete if it occurs in the first 2 to 3 years of life, but afterward, there is risk of laryngeal muscle atrophy, cricoarytenoid fixation, and/or synkinesis, which will result in incomplete vocal fold motion.[21]

Some children with unilateral paralysis will require vocal fold injection to prevent aspiration with feeds and improve dysphonia, but this is not typically the case in patients with respiratory symptoms. In patients with bilateral paralysis and respiratory distress, vocal fold lateralization, cricoid split, or tracheotomy may be necessary to create a definitive airway within the first few weeks of life. When the child is older and tracheotomy is no longer needed for ventilation purposes, both static (posterior cricoid graft, lateral cordotomy, arytenoidectomy) and dynamic (vocal fold reinnervation with muscle pedicle or ansa cervicalis-to-recurrent laryngeal nerve grafting) surgery can be offered to widen the glottic aperture.[21]

Subglottic Stenosis

Biphasic stridor can be significant for subglottic stenosis, a narrowing of the trachea just below the vocal cords at the level of the cricoid cartilage. Children typically present with stridor, cough, and recurrent croup. For example, a low-pitched barky cough that acutely develops during a viral illness may signal an underlying subglottic pathologic condition. Subglottic stenosis is more commonly acquired secondary to long-term intubation or trauma but can also present as a congenital abnormality, and it requires a direct laryngoscopy with bronchoscopy for definitive diagnosis. Acquired lesions are typically more severe than congenital subglottic narrowing, and concomitant lesions can be discovered on bronchoscopy.[4] Depending on symptoms, tracheostomy may be necessary if respiratory distress persists. Endoscopic management with balloon dilation and laser excision of stenosis may prevent need for tracheotomy and further airway surgery. However, open airway reconstruction is typically the definitive treatment in patients who have failed previous management or have narrowed segments too severe for endoscopic therapy.

Laryngeal Web

Stridor at birth can also be secondary to a laryngeal web/partial atresia, a rare congenital anomaly secondary to failure of the embryonic glottic airway to recanalize. This condition occurs on a spectrum of severity, extending from thin membranous webs that can be lysed versus thick cartilaginous webs resulting from laryngeal atresia.[31] The disorder can also be associated with genetic conditions, such as DiGeorge syndrome. Most laryngeal webs are anterior in location partially affecting motion of the vocal cords. Patients present with voice disorder or stridor during the neonatal period.

Depending on severity, endoscopic lysis of the laryngeal web or open reconstruction is an effective treatment. Severe cases of laryngeal atresia may require an ex utero intrapartum treatment procedure to secure an airway with a tracheotomy upon birth.

Laryngeal Cleft and Tracheoesophageal Fistulas

Stridor secondary to laryngeal cleft is rare, with an incidence of less than 0.1%.[32] The condition develops as an incomplete partition of the tracheoesophageal septum, resulting in a communication of the posterior larynx and esophagus. The condition can be present in isolation or can be associated with several syndromes, including Opitz-Frias, Pallister-Hall, and VACTERL. There are multiple classification schemes of the laryngeal cleft, all based on the length of the incomplete partition. The Benjamin-Ingles scale is one such classification system, where the laryngeal cleft extends deep into the interarytenoid space above the vocal cords (type I), into the cricoid cartilage (type II), through the cricoid cartilage (type III), and into the intrathoracic tracheoesophageal wall (type IV).[33] Symptoms correlate with the length of the cleft, but some children can be asymptomatic. Children with symptomatic disease will have inspiratory stridor, cyanosis, aspiration, and recurrent pneumonia episodes. The diagnosis is suspected by flexible fiber-optic laryngoscopy and documented by direct laryngoscopy with bronchoscopy, with particular attention to palpation of the interarytenoid area. A modified barium swallow study not only supports the endoscopic diagnosis but also objectively assesses aspiration. Children with a small type I laryngeal cleft are treated initially with conservative management, including improved feeding positioning, acid reflux control, and liquid thickener in feeds. In patients who have failed conservative management or who have pulmonary sequalae, augmentation with interarytenoid injection or definitive surgical repair, depending on size of the cleft, is recommended.[34] Clefts extending to or through the cricoid (types II, III, and IV) will require surgical repair.

Tracheoesophageal fistula (TEF) is the most common congenital anomaly affecting the esophagus when presenting with esophageal atresia (EA). Like laryngeal clefts, TEF also presents as an isolated incomplete partition of the tracheoesophageal septum. There are 5 types of anomalies, with the most common subtype being a distal tracheal fistula with EA (type III), followed by isolated EA without TEF, H-type TEF, EA with proximal TEF, and EA with both proximal and distal TEF.[35] Most patients will present shortly after birth because of the inability to pass a 10F catheter beyond 10 cm in the setting of drooling, respiratory distress, or cyanosis with feeds.[35] Plain chest radiographs will reveal the presence or absence of a gastric bubble depending on the presence of EA with or without TEF, in addition to coiling of a nasogastric tube in patients with EA. Contrast studies are rarely required, owing to risk of pneumonitis, and direct laryngoscopy with bronchoscopy is useful in this setting for visualization of fistula. The condition can be present in isolation or associated with several syndromes, including CHARGE and VACTERL. Treatment involves placement of a gastrostomy tube for definitive feeding management, with repair of the fistula by 3 months of age.[35] Repair can be performed endoscopically or with open repair with esophageal anastomosis and fistula closure.

Tracheomalacia

Tracheomalacia is a dynamic anomaly of the upper-respiratory tract owing to abnormal weakness of the tracheal walls and supporting cartilage (**Fig. 6**). The condition can be a primary condition, typically owing to gestational prematurity resulting in flattened and shorter tracheal cartilage, or secondary to underlying vascular compression, TEF, relapsing polychondritis, or Ehlers-Danlos syndrome. Tracheomalacia can

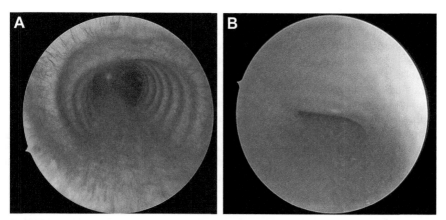

Fig. 6. Appearance of normal distal trachea (*A*) and severe tracheomalacia (*B*).

also be acquired owing to longstanding intubation trauma or subsequent tracheotomy, which can weaken tracheal cartilage. Collapse of the tracheal cartilage can lead to barking cough, frequent respiratory infections, and cyanotic episodes. Definitive diagnosis is necessary with rigid endoscopy or tracheoscopy to visualize dynamic collapse of the airway in an anteroposterior fashion. Treatment is typically conservative management and continuous positive pressure ventilation in the setting of tracheostomy tube placement.[35] Most infants will improve within 6 to 12 months of age as the cartilage develops, but the condition can be long-lasting and worsen with age depending on the underlying cause.[1] In severe cases of vascular compression resulting in tracheomalacia, anterior aortopexy or posterior tracheopexy is necessary to resolve airway obstruction. Placement of a tracheostomy tube or distal airway stent can be used in refractory disease but should be avoided because of the high likelihood of permanent tracheal damage. They are to be used in urgent or emergent conditions in patients whose prognosis is unlikely to improve without open surgical intervention.[35]

Complete Tracheal Rings

Complete tracheal rings are a birth defect secondary to abnormal growth of the cartilage during gestation. In a normally developed trachea, the cartilage distal to the cricoid is in a C-shaped ring with trachealis muscle forming the posterior border. A trachea with complete rings will have rigid O-shaped rings throughout the length of the trachea, resulting in a narrowed airway. The condition is typically associated with cardiovascular anomalies, Down syndrome, or Pfeiffer syndrome. Children will present with noisy breathing, stridor, wheezing, apnea, and recurrent pneumonia. Diagnosis is with rigid endoscopy and imaging (CT scan or MRI scan). Mild presentation can be watched conservatively until definitive management may be necessary. Children with severe presentation will require definitive surgery, such as tracheal resection or slide tracheoplasty. Because of the high likelihood of concomitant cardiovascular anomalies, these procedures should be performed alongside cardiovascular surgery.

Infectious Stridor

Stridor of an infectious cause is not typically seen in the neonatal or infant age group and is more common in older children. However, when stridor presents acutely, the most common cause is laryngotracheobronchitis, or croup.[36] Croup causes subglottic edema, which results in an expiratory barking cough along with an inspiratory stridor.

Patients will also have low-grade fever with negative blood cultures and normal white blood cell counts. Radiographic evaluation will show subglottic narrowing. The condition presents mostly in children 6 to 24 months of age and usually is preceded by an upper-respiratory infection. Therapy is mostly supportive care with humidification and nebulized racemic epinephrine. Children with recurrent croup in the setting of repeated hospitalizations and history of endotracheal intubation should undergo workup by an otolaryngologist for underlying anatomic abnormality.[4]

Epiglottitis is another bacterial inflammation of the larynx, typically caused by *Haemophilus influenzae* type B, that usually occurs in children 3 to 6 years of age during the winter season. Thankfully, the incidence of epiglottitis in children has been reduced dramatically because of the widespread use of the *H influenzae* vaccine and is rarely seen in the neonatal age group.[4,28,37]

Foreign Body

Although not a congenital condition, foreign body obstruction should be considered an acute cause of stridor. Aspiration is most common between the ages of 1 to 3 years old. Foreign body obstruction in the postcricoid space and esophagus can also result in airway compromise owing to tracheal compression, typically producing a biphasic stridor. Patient history typically follows an episode of choking after placement of food or foreign body in the mouth, followed by gagging or wheezing alongside hoarseness, stridor, or complete airway obstruction. In situations of unwitnessed aspiration or mild symptoms, a delayed presentation may occur with cough, fevers, malaise, and signs of pneumonia. Definitive treatment involves operative extraction with direct laryngoscopy and rigid bronchoscopy.

MANAGEMENT OF LARYNGOMALACIA
Conservative Management

Laryngomalacia resolves with conservative management for most children, and the vast majority will not need operative intervention. Routine follow-up to monitor symptoms is adequate to prevent adverse developments, such as worsening stridor or BRUEs. Most patients will improve in some fashion before 12 to 18 months of age.

Medications to manage acid reflux have been helpful in conservative management.[34] Acid suppression therapy, consisting of either a histamine receptor blocker or a proton-pump inhibitor, has been linked to improved stridor, reduced respiratory distress, and a shorter symptom course.[5,10] Recently, safety concerns regarding the link of acid reflux medication to cancer and dementia have arisen in the literature, but studies linking short courses of the medication with adverse effects in children have not been established.[38,39] Discussions with both the parent and the primary care provider should occur before starting acid reflux medication for long-term treatment of laryngomalacia owing to these safety concerns. At the time of this writing, famotidine has been the therapy of choice for treatment of children with reflux.

Surgical Treatment

Up to 10% of children with laryngomalacia will require surgical management because of severe disease. If not treated promptly, complications, such as apnea, feeding difficulties and failure to thrive, cor pulmonale, and even death, may occur owing to untreated respiratory obstruction. Historically, these children were treated with tracheotomy for most of the twentieth century, and this procedure may still be necessary depending on there being an underlying neurologic component.[4]

Over the last 36 years, supraglottoplasty has become the surgical treatment of choice for laryngomalacia (**Fig. 7**). The basic principles of this procedure have evolved over time, but the treatment addresses the redundant tissue along the 3 components of laryngomalacia: the epiglottis, aryepiglottic folds, and arytenoids.[16] Patients are placed under general anesthesia for the procedure, typically at the same time as a diagnostic direct laryngoscopy with bronchoscopy. After confirmation of no serious synchronous airway lesions, surgery can be performed with the patient breathing spontaneously. In patients with poor pulmonary reserve, intubation is sometimes necessary, although this can interfere with surgical exposure of the larynx.

Many surgical procedures were contemplated over the past 120 years. Variot[40] in 1898 suggested excision of the aryepiglottic folds to relieve laryngomalacia-based obstruction but never performed the procedure, as his theories were based on a post-mortem examination of a baby. Epiglottopexy, or the suturing of the epiglottis to the base of tongue, was described by Fearon and Ellis[41] in 1971 as a treatment for the ret-roflexed epiglottis. This technique has fallen out of favor for lack of good outcomes.

Seid and colleagues[42] described cutting the aryepiglottic fold for all cases of laryng-omalacia, which also had limited success. Cold technique laryngoplasty was first described by Zalzal and colleagues[16] in 1987. In this technique, cold steel instruments are used to divide the aryepiglottic folds, trim the lateral edges of the epiglottis, and resect redundant supra-arytenoid mucosa, depending on which area or areas were causing obstruction. Use of CO_2 laser later became a common procedure as well.[42,43] Microdebrider-based supraglottoplasty was first described in 2005 by Zalzal and Collins[44] as an additional tool in combination with the classic cold technique supraglottoplasty (Video 1). The suction component of the microdebrider resects redundant tissue and clears blood from the laryngeal field in this technique, which al-lows for a clean plane of dissection of the excess supraglottic tissue following incision of the aryepiglottic fold.[45]

Recently, coblation technology has been used as another tool for operative supra-glottoplasty as a safer alternative to CO_2 laser excision, as the risk of airway fires is much less.[43] However, there have not been many outcomes studies using this method over the last decade, and more research is still needed on its feasibility as a laser alternative.[46]

Surgical Outcomes and Complications

Overall, success rates following supraglottoplasty range up to 95%.[47] Failures are either due to technical errors, such as conservative resection of redundant supraglottic

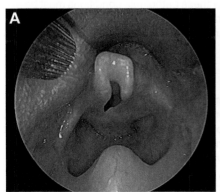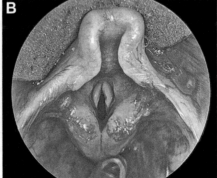

Fig. 7. Supraglottoplasty images, before (*A*) and after (*B*) repair of laryngomalacia.

mucosa or epiglottic cartilage, or to inherent patient characteristics. A systemic review by Preciado and Zalzal[46] found that failure in infants is significantly associated with children with neurologic and medical comorbidities compared with those without.

Complications following supraglottoplasty are rare, but include aspiration, supraglottic stenosis, cartilage damage, airway fires, and granuloma formation.[5] Inflammation and airway edema are transient issues that may develop in the immediate postoperative period but can be controlled with an adequate postoperative medication regimen. The most serious complication, supraglottic stenosis, is a rare occurrence that will require repeat operative resection of scarring and monitoring to prevent further narrowing of the airway.

POSTOPERATIVE MANAGEMENT

Practice management for children who undergo surgical treatment for laryngomalacia involves multiple factors. In 2016, a survey of 101 otolaryngologists who perform supraglottoplasty shared their strategies for postsupraglottoplasty care. Most patients will receive perioperative steroids to help with postoperative laryngeal edema, with several undergoing a taper of steroids for several days postoperatively.[43] Depending on physician preference, antibiotics are prescribed postoperatively, with most who do prescribe antibiotics given at least 5 days of medical therapy.[43] Regarding acid suppression therapy, the International Pediatric Otolaryngology Group published postoperative guidelines recommending that proton-pump inhibition or histamine-2 receptor antagonists should be continued for at least 3 months postoperatively.[34]

Children should be monitored for at least 24 hours postoperatively in the event laryngeal edema worsens in that timeframe. Patient monitoring should ideally take place in a recovery room or intensive care unit setting. Nearly all patients will leave the hospital the following morning if there are no desaturation events or feeding difficulties postoperatively.

Swallowing outcomes should not be affected after the procedure if performed correctly. Patients correct immediately after the procedure. Should there be a concern for dysphagia or aspiration after the procedure, evaluation by speech therapy or evaluation with flexible endoscopy can be performed before discharge. Routine follow-up is performed within 4 to 6 weeks of the operation to confirm resolution of symptoms.[34] Repeat flexible endoscopy in clinic does not need to be performed if there is no clinical indication for the procedure. Depending on the reason for the initial consultation, both swallowing and breathing outcomes should improve by the first postoperative visit. If the patient continues to have respiratory noise when breathing or if signs of failure to thrive are still present, alternative causes for these pathologic conditions must be evaluated. This may include need for repeat direct laryngoscopy with bronchoscopy, or alternative workup for failure to thrive and swallowing dysfunction in conjunction with the patient's primary care provider.

SUMMARY

Stridor presents as an inspiratory, expiratory, or biphasic noise owing to obstruction or narrowing somewhere along the respiratory tract. Diagnosis is dependent on visualization of the airway, typically by flexible fiber-optic laryngoscopy in the clinic or direct laryngoscopy with bronchoscopy under anesthesia. In some cases, a barium swallow study will be needed to evaluate cause. Laryngomalacia is the most common cause of inspiratory stridor in neonates and infants, with 10% of children having severe symptoms requiring surgical intervention. Supraglottoplasty will result in good outcomes for most children with laryngomalacia.

CLINICS CARE POINTS

- When evaluating a child with stridor, identify duration and severity of the underlying respiratory distress when gathering a history.
- Physical examination should focus on the quality of the stridor being produced in addition to signs of respiratory distress, such as tracheal tugging or sternal retraction.
- In the stable patient, the gold standard to evaluating the stridulous child is laryngeal examination with endoscopy.
- In the unstable patient, evaluation of the airway under anesthesia with direct laryngoscopy and bronchoscopy is preferred before intubation, if possible.
- Chronic stridor most commonly is secondary to laryngomalacia, in which operative intervention should be performed in patients showing symptoms of failure to thrive.

SUPPLEMENTARY DATA

Supplementary data related to this article can be found online at https://doi.org/10.1016/j.pcl.2021.12.003.

REFERENCES

1. Claes J, Boudewyns A, Deron P, et al. Management of stridor in neonates and infants. B-ENT 2005;(Suppl 1):113–22 [quiz: 23–5].
2. Caussade Larraín S, Flores Berríos C. Children with persistent stridor. In: Bertrand Pablo, Sanchez Ignacio, editors. Pediatric respiratory diseases. Cham, Switzerland: Springer; 2020. p. 193–9.
3. Monnier P. Clinical evaluation of airway obstruction. In: Monnier P, editor. Pediatric airway surgery. Berlin: Springer; 2011. p. 31–44.
4. Zalzal GH. Stridor and airway compromise. Pediatr Clin North Am 1989;36(6): 1389–402.
5. Bedwell J, Zalzal G. Laryngomalacia. Semin Pediatr Surg 2016;25(3):119–22.
6. Holinger LD. Etiology of stridor in the neonate, infant and child. Ann Otol Rhinol Laryngol 1980;89(5 Pt 1):397–400.
7. Zoumalan R, Maddalozzo J, Holinger LD. Etiology of stridor in infants. Ann Otol Rhinol Laryngol 2007;116(5):329–34.
8. Barthez E, Rilliet F. Traité clinique et pratique des maladies des enfants. Paris: Germer Baillière; 1853.
9. Belmont JR, Grundfast K. Congenital laryngeal stridor (laryngomalacia): etiologic factors and associated disorders. Ann Otol Rhinol Laryngol 1984;93(5 Pt 1): 430–7.
10. Thompson DM. Abnormal sensorimotor integrative function of the larynx in congenital laryngomalacia: a new theory of etiology. Laryngoscope 2007;117(6 Pt 2 Suppl 114):1–33.
11. Olney DR, Greinwald JH Jr, Smith RJ, et al. Laryngomalacia and its treatment. Laryngoscope 1999;109(11):1770–5.
12. Simons JP, Greenberg LL, Mehta DK, et al. Laryngomalacia and swallowing function in children. Laryngoscope 2016;126(2):478–84.
13. Dickson JM, Richter GT, Meinzen-Derr J, et al. Secondary airway lesions in infants with laryngomalacia. Ann Otol Rhinol Laryngol 2009;118(1):37–43.

14. Mancuso RF, Choi SS, Zalzal GH, et al. Laryngomalacia. The search for the second lesion. Arch Otolaryngol Head Neck Surg 1996;122(3):302–6.
15. Schroeder JW Jr, Bhandarkar ND, Holinger LD. Synchronous airway lesions and outcomes in infants with severe laryngomalacia requiring supraglottoplasty. Arch Otolaryngol Head Neck Surg 2009;135(7):647–51.
16. Zalzal GH, Anon JB, Cotton RT. Epiglottoplasty for the treatment of laryngomalacia. Ann Otol Rhinol Laryngol 1987;96(1 Pt 1):72–6.
17. Berg E, Naseri I, Sobol SE. The role of airway fluoroscopy in the evaluation of children with stridor. Arch Otolaryngol Head Neck Surg 2008;134(4):415–8.
18. Orlow SJ, Isakoff MS, Blei F. Increased risk of symptomatic hemangiomas of the airway in association with cutaneous hemangiomas in a "beard" distribution. J Pediatr 1997;131(4):643–6.
19. Tunkel DE, Zalzal GH. Stridor in infants and children: ambulatory evaluation and operative diagnosis. Clin Pediatr (Phila) 1992;31(1):48–55.
20. Peridis S, Pilgrim G, Athanasopoulos I, et al. A meta-analysis on the effectiveness of propranolol for the treatment of infantile airway haemangiomas. Int J Pediatr Otorhinolaryngol 2011;75(4):455–60.
21. Siddel D, Mesner A. Evaluation and management of the pediatric airway. In: Flint PWHB, Lund VJ, editors. Cummings otolaryngology-head and neck surgery 3. 7th edition. Philadelphia: Elsevier; 2020. p. 3053–67.
22. Lim J, Hellier W, Harcourt J, et al. Subglottic cysts: the Great Ormond Street experience. Int J Pediatr Otorhinolaryngol 2003;67(5):461–5.
23. Best SR, Friedman AD, Landau-Zemer T, et al. Safety and dosing of bevacizumab (Avastin) for the treatment of recurrent respiratory papillomatosis. Ann Otol Rhinol Laryngol 2012;121(9):587–93.
24. Best SR, Mohr M, Zur KB. Systemic bevacizumab for recurrent respiratory papillomatosis: a national survey. Laryngoscope 2017;127(10):2225–9.
25. Novakovic D, Cheng ATL, Zurynski Y, et al. A prospective study of the incidence of juvenile-onset recurrent respiratory papillomatosis after implementation of a national HPV vaccination program. J Infect Dis 2018;217(2):208–12.
26. Petrosky E, Bocchini JA Jr, Hariri S, et al. Use of 9-valent human papillomavirus (HPV) vaccine: updated HPV vaccination recommendations of the advisory committee on immunization practices. MMWR Morb Mortal Wkly Rep 2015; 64(11):300.
27. Holinger LD, Holinger PC, Holinger PH. Etiology of bilateral abductor vocal cord paralysis: a review of 389 cases. Ann Otol Rhinol Laryngol 1976;85(4 Pt 1): 428–36.
28. Leung AK, Cho H. Diagnosis of stridor in children. Am Fam Physician 1999;60(8): 2289–96.
29. de Gaudemar I, Roudaire M, François M, et al. Outcome of laryngeal paralysis in neonates: a long term retrospective study of 113 cases. Int J Pediatr Otorhinolaryngol 1996;34(1–2):101–10.
30. Miyamoto RC, Parikh SR, Gellad W, et al. Bilateral congenital vocal cord paralysis: a 16-year institutional review. Otolaryngol Head Neck Surg 2005;133(2): 241–5.
31. Cohen SR. Congenital glottic webs in children. A retrospective review of 51 patients. Ann Otol Rhinol Laryngol Suppl 1985;121:2–16.
32. Pezzettigotta SM, Leboulanger N, Roger G, et al. Laryngeal cleft. Otolaryngol Clin North Am 2008;41(5):913–33, ix.
33. Benjamin B, Inglis A. Minor congenital laryngeal clefts: diagnosis and classification. Ann Otol Rhinol Laryngol 1989;98(6):417–20.

34. Carter J, Rahbar R, Brigger M, et al. International Pediatric ORL Group (IPOG) laryngomalacia consensus recommendations. Int J Pediatr Otorhinolaryngol 2016;86:256–61.
35. Green G, Ohye R. Diagnosis and management of tracheal anomalies and tracheal stenosis. In: Flint PWHB, Lund VJ, editors. Cummings otolaryngology-head and neck surgery 3. 7th edition. Philadelphia: Elsevier; 2020. p. 3107–18.
36. Sobol SE, Zapata S. Epiglottitis and croup. Otolaryngol Clin North Am 2008;41(3): 551–66, ix.
37. Allen M, Meraj TS, Oska S, et al. Acute epiglottitis: analysis of U.S. mortality trends from 1979 to 2017. Am J Otolaryngol 2021;42(2):102882.
38. Fallahzadeh MK, Borhani Haghighi A, Namazi MR. Proton pump inhibitors: predisposers to Alzheimer disease? J Clin Pharm Ther 2010;35(2):125–6.
39. Mahase E. FDA recalls ranitidine medicines over potential cancer causing impurity. BMJ 2019;367:l5832.
40. Variot G. Un cas de respiration stridoreuse des nouveau-nes avec autopsie. Bull Mem Soc Med Hop Paris 1898;3:490–4.
41. Fearon B, Ellis D. The management of long term airway problems in infants and children. Ann Otol Rhinol Laryngol 1971;80(5):669–77.
42. Seid AB, Park SM, Kearns MJ, et al. Laser division of the aryepiglottic folds for severe laryngomalacia. Int J Pediatr Otorhinolaryngol 1985;10(2):153–8.
43. Ramprasad VH, Ryan MA, Farjat AE, et al. Practice patterns in supraglottoplasty and perioperative care. Int J Pediatr Otorhinolaryngol 2016;86:118–23.
44. Zalzal GH, Collins WO. Microdebrider-assisted supraglottoplasty. Int J Pediatr Otorhinolaryngol 2005;69(3):305–9.
45. Groblewski JC, Shah RK, Zalzal GH. Microdebrider-assisted supraglottoplasty for laryngomalacia. Ann Otol Rhinol Laryngol 2009;118(8):592–7.
46. Preciado D, Zalzal G. A systematic review of supraglottoplasty outcomes. Arch Otolaryngol Head Neck Surg 2012;138(8):718–21.
47. Reddy DK, Matt BH. Unilateral vs. bilateral supraglottoplasty for severe laryngomalacia in children. Arch Otolaryngol Head Neck Surg 2001;127(6):694–9.

Recurrent Croup

Huma Quraishi, MD[a], Donna J. Lee, MD[a,*]

KEYWORDS

- Recurrent croup • Croup • Stridor • Spasmodic croup

KEY POINTS

- Recurrent croup is a symptom rather than a distinct disease.
- Recurrent croup warrants a work-up for an underlying cause.
- Causes associated with recurrent croup include:
  - Airway abnormality
  - Atopic airway disease, such as asthma
  - Gastroesophageal reflux (GERD)
- Airway abnormality is often found in patients with recurrent croup before 1 year of age, with history of intubation, and severe presentation that warrant hospital admission.
- Work-up should be performed by a multidisciplinary team.
- Consider antiasthma and/or anti-GERD treatment in patients without strong suspicion for airway abnormality.

Croup, or laryngotracheobronchitis, refers to airway inflammation and edema leading to obstruction of the larynx, trachea, and bronchi often as a result of viral infection and is the most common cause of acute airway obstruction in young children. It is characterized by the onset of low-grade fever, barky cough, stridor, hoarseness, and a variable degree of respiratory distress. Croup is typically preceded by 24 to 48 hours of nasal congestion and rhinorrhea. Parainfluenza is the most common cause of viral or infectious croup; however, infection with multiple other respiratory viruses can also result in croup. Viral croup typically occurs between 6 months and 3 years of age, with a peak at 18 months. Croup symptoms typically resolve within 48 hours but may last up to a week.[1,2]

Croup can also occur in the absence of a viral prodrome. The term spasmodic croup has been used to describe this scenario to differentiate it from viral croup. Patients are typically well and then develop sudden onset of barky cough and stridor at night.

Funding Sources: None.
Conflict of Interest: None.
[a] Division of Pediatric Pulmonology, Joseph M. Sanzari Children's Hospital, Hackensack Meridian Children's Health, 30 Prospect Avenue, WFAN PC377, Hackensack, NJ 07601, USA
* Corresponding author.
E-mail address: donna.lee@hmhn.org

Pediatr Clin N Am 69 (2022) 319–328
https://doi.org/10.1016/j.pcl.2021.12.004
0031-3955/22/© 2021 Elsevier Inc. All rights reserved.

Spasmodic croup typically occurs in older children, has a rapid onset and a rapid resolution, and often has a recurrent course. The cause of spasmodic croup is unclear. Allergy, airway hyperreactivity, and gastroesophageal reflux have all been implicated as possible causative factors. One unproven theory is that spasmodic croup may be an allergic reaction to viral antigen rather than direct infection.[3,4]

Recurrent croup, viral or spasmodic, has been defined many ways but the most accepted definition is two or more episodes per year. Van Bever and coworkers[5] estimated recurrent viral croup (defined as >3 episode) has an incidence of 5%. When recurrent croup occurs it should be considered a symptom of an underlying airway abnormality, either structural or inflammatory, and should prompt a work-up for the underlying cause.

STRUCTURAL AIRWAY ABNORMALITY

Recurrent croup may be the first manifestation of an underlying congenital or acquired airway abnormality (**Box 1**). Even though viral croup results from inflammation throughout the airway, the subglottis is the primary site of airway obstruction. The subglottis is bounded by the cricoid cartilage and is the narrowest portion of the pediatric airway. Because the cricoid is the only complete cartilaginous ring in the airway, there is no room for outward expansion with edema or inflammation. One millimeter of circumferential swelling can significantly reduce the area and airflow within the normal pediatric airway (**Fig. 1**). The incidence of croup declines after 3 years of age because the caliber of the airway has grown sufficiently to withstand compromise from viral inflammation. However, if a child has an underlying narrowing of the airway, they may be susceptible to developing croup with even mild airway inflammation from a

---

Box 1
Causes of recurrent croup

- Anatomic
  - Glottic
    - Vocal cord paralysis/paresis
    - Laryngomalacia
    - Laryngeal web
  - Subglottic
    - Congenital or acquired stenosis
    - Subglottic hemangioma
    - Subglottic cyst
  - Tracheal
    - Tracheobronchomalacia
    - Complete tracheal ring
    - Tracheal stenosis
    - Tracheoesophageal fistula
  - Extrinsic compression
    - Vascular ring
    - Innominate artery compression
    - Mediastinal mass
  - Other
    - Retained foreign body

- Functional
  - Asthma
  - Gastroesophageal reflux disease
  - Eosinophilic esophagitis

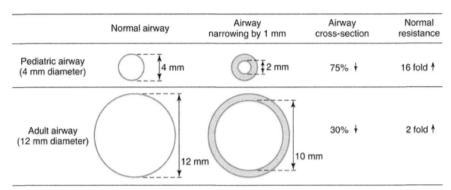

	Normal airway	Airway narrowing by 1 mm	Airway cross-section	Normal resistance
Pediatric airway (4 mm diameter)	4 mm	2 mm	75% ↓	16 fold ↑
Adult airway (12 mm diameter)	12 mm	10 mm	30% ↓	2 fold ↑

Fig. 1. Schematic diagram demonstrating why minor narrowing in a child's airway is of much greater consequence than in an adult. For example, 1 mm of edema in a 4-mm diameter pediatric airway reduces the cross-sectional area by 75% (16-fold increase in resistance), whereas in a 12-mm adult airway, the same 1 mm of edema reduces the airway area by just 30% (two-fold increase in resistance). Calculation is based on Poiseuille's law, the principles of tubular flow, $Q = [\pi r4(P1-P2)]/8\eta L$; where Q is flow, r is radius, P is pressure, η is viscosity, and L is length of tube. This law indicates that resistance is inversely proportional to the radius to the fourth power. (Reprint with permission from Ento Key: evaluation-and-management-of-the-stridulous-child.)

viral upper respiratory tract infection. Furthermore, the onset of croup may be earlier than 6 months, more severe in presentation, and may continue to occur beyond 3 years of age.[3]

Several studies have examined the incidence of airway abnormalities in children with recurrent croup.[6–10] Subglottic stenosis was most commonly identified in 30.6% of cases, followed by tracheomalacia in 4.6%. Vocal cord pathology, subglottic cysts and hemangiomas, and retained foreign bodies were less frequently encountered.[11] Most cases of subglottic stenosis were mild and did not require any further treatment. Only 5% to 10% of children were found to have more severe forms of stenosis requiring surgical intervention.[6,7,9,10]

Several factors have been found to correlate with a positive finding of an airway abnormality on bronchoscopy. Multiple studies have identified onset of recurrent croup at less than 3 years of age as a risk factor for an underlying airway abnormality.[6,9,10,12] Jabbour[7] identified age less than 1 year at presentation to be predictive of a moderate to severe airway abnormality. A prior history of intubation and prematurity also correlated with a finding of airway abnormality on bronchoscopy. This is not surprising because they are also risk factors for acquired subglottic stenosis. Lastly, those patients that received an inpatient consultation from otolaryngology, indicating the severity of the episode, were also more likely to have an underlying airway abnormality.

One study identified the presence of chronic cough as a risk factor for abnormal findings on bronchoscopy. This study included signs of gastroesophageal reflux disease (GERD) as an abnormal finding in addition to structural abnormalities. GERD has been associated with chronic cough. Eleven percent of patients in this study were found to have tracheomalacia.[12] Tracheomalacia is defined as an increased collapsibility of the airway either from intrinsic causes, such as increased laxity of the posterior membranous trachea or impaired cartilage integrity, or as a result of extrinsic external compression, such as from a vascular ring, innominate artery, or mediastinal masses.[13] Airway narrowing is most apparent on expiration and presents as expiratory stridor and a barky cough. The barky cough is thought to occur from contact of the anterior and posterior walls of the trachea resulting in recurrent vibrations.[14] Tracheomalacia can present with a recurrent or chronic barky cough that is exacerbated by viral infection and may be misdiagnosed as recurrent croup.

Several factors were not associated with airway abnormalities on bronchoscopy. These include a history of allergy, GERD, and the number of episodes of croup. Interestingly, two studies found that there was no significant difference in the presence of airway abnormalities in the children who presented with spasmodic croup compared with those that had a viral prodrome.[4]

KEY POINTS

- Any child presenting with recurrent croup before 1 year of age should undergo bronchoscopy to rule out an underlying airway abnormality.
- Bronchoscopy should be considered in children presenting with recurrent croup before 3 years of age.
- Bronchoscopy should be considered in children presenting with recurrent croup who have a prior history of intubation.
- Bronchoscopy should be considered in children presenting with recurrent croup who required hospital admission.

GASTROESOPHAGEAL REFLUX DISEASE

Up to 50% of patients with recurrent croup also have GERD.[15] Recurrent croup has been postulated to be an extraesophageal manifestation of GERD. GERD has been shown to be a risk factor for subglottic stenosis; however, a history of GERD did not correlate with the presence of airway narrowing on endoscopy.[11,16,17] Another possible explanation is that microaspiration into the upper airway may contribute to damage to the mucosal barrier and result in an increased susceptibility to viral infection.[18]

The current literature supports an association between recurrent croup and GERD but a causal relationship has not been established. One of the challenges is that there is no universally accepted modality to diagnose GERD. Radiologic studies, pH probe, bronchoalveolar lavage, and esophagoscopy with biopsy have all been used in published studies. Furthermore, several studies have relied on bronchoscopy findings of posterior glottic erythema and edema, subglottic edema, tracheal cobblestoning or folliculitis, and blunting of the carina as signs of GERD.[8,19–21]

In a retrospective study of 235 children with recurrent croup, Duval[19] reported that tracheal folliculitis was present in 41% of patients. The cause of tracheal folliculitis is unclear but is believed to be an inflammatory response to aspiration, allergy, and/or GERD. A subset of 117 patients in this study also had objective diagnostic testing for GERD by 24-hour pH probe, barium swallow, and/or esophageal biopsies. No significant difference was found in the incidence of tracheal folliculitis in children who had GERD (43.5%) on objective testing compared with those who did not have GERD (37.5%).

There was also no correlation between the diagnosis of GERD and the presence of subglottic or arytenoid edema.[19,21] This suggests that tracheal folliculitis and airway edema are nonspecific signs of inflammation rather than signs of GERD. Another possible explanation is that this study reflects the limitations of the previously mentioned modalities in accurately diagnosing GERD.

Krishnan and coworkers[22] have suggested that testing tracheal secretions obtained from bronchoscopy for the presence of pepsin may provide a more accurate assessment for GERD-related respiratory disease. In a study of 118 children, 98 of whom had recurrent croup, a positive pepsin assay was found to correlate with a history of recurrent croup. A positive pepsin assay did not correlate with a previous diagnosis of GERD by standard testing modalities.[22]

The most compelling evidence for GERD as a contributing factor to recurrent croup is that multiple studies have shown an improvement in the severity and frequency of episodes of croup with treatment of GERD.[18,20,21] Hoa[21] reported on 35 patients with findings consistent with GERD on bronchoscopy that were treated with ranitidine and metoclopramide, a motility agent. Thirty-one out of the 35 patients (89%) experienced an improvement in the severity, duration, and frequency of croup episodes. However, 45% still continued to have some symptoms. Seventy-six percent and 90% improvement were also found in patients treated for GERD as reported by Kwong and coworkers[20] and Rankin and coworkers,[8] respectively. The results of these studies suggest that patients who have signs of inflammation in the airway on laryngobronchoscopy will benefit from treatment with antireflux medications.

KEY POINTS

- Treatment of GERD can result in improvement in the severity and frequency of episodes of recurrent croup.

ATOPIC CONDITIONS
Asthma

Atopy is defined as the genetic tendency to develop allergic diseases with a heightened immune response to ingested or inhaled allergens. Manifestations of atopy can occur on skin (eczema) and in the aerodigestive tract (allergic rhinitis, asthma, and eosinophilic esophagitis [EoE]).[23] Asthma is an atopic disease characterized by chronic airway inflammation with airway hyperresponsiveness/hyperreactivity as the hallmark feature. Airway hyperreactivity is the tendency for bronchoconstriction in response to various agents including histamine, methacholine, and exercise.[24,25]

Speculation for the association between recurrent croup and atopic conditions was based on several observational studies that revealed a higher incidence of recurrent croup in patients with atopy or a family history of atopy.[26,27] Zach and colleagues[28] reported that recurrent croup is more prevalent in patients that have a history of allergies, have lower expiratory flow rates on pulmonary function testing, and have increased airway hyperreactivity/hyperresponsiveness. In this study, patients with recurrent croup were more likely to go on to develop asthma.

In a random sampling of 5756 Belgian children, recurrent coup was also found to be strongly associated with a diagnosis of asthma, wheezing, and the use of antiasthma medications. However, no significant difference was found on skin prick testing to various aeroallergens in patients without croup, with croup, and with recurrent croup. A family history of asthma was also not associated with either croup or recurrent croup. However, a family history of other atopic disease (eczema, allergic rhinitis, chronic bronchitis) was found to be associated with croup and strongly associated with recurrent croup. Assessment of pulmonary function revealed that children with croup had lower expiratory flow rates compared with children without croup. This study found that recurrent croup is associated with a history of asthma but not aeroallergen sensitization, concluding that asthma is a result of small airway caliber, rather than environmental allergy.[5] However, a large prospective study investigating the onset of asthma in children did not support this conclusion. Croup was not found to be a predictor of asthma in later life.[29]

KEY POINTS

- Although there is an association between croup and atopy, this relationship is complex.
- Recurrent croup may be associated with development of asthma later in life.
- A direct causal relationship between recurrent croup and atopy/asthma was not identified.

EOSINOPHILIC ESOPHAGITIS

EoE is a well-documented disease entity in pediatric patients. Patients often present to pediatric gastroenterologists with esophageal dysfunction, food impaction, GERD, and dysphagia resulting in failure to thrive. The hallmark of EoE is chronic inflammation with eosinophil infiltration of the esophagus. Patients with EoE have a high propensity for personal and family history of atopy.[30] Diagnosis of EoE requires presence of significant eosinophilia (>15 eosinophils per high powered field) on esophageal biopsy. Although most patients present with gastrointestinal complaints, there is a growing body of literature reporting upper airway complaints, such as dysphonia, cough, stridor, and recurrent croup in patients who were found to have EoE.[31–33] These patients with airway complaints presented to otolaryngology at an earlier age compared with patients who presented to gastroenterology. Cooper and coworkers[34] reviewed 85 surgical charts of patients who underwent endoscopy for atypical croup or recurrent croup. Evidence of esophagitis was found in 36 children, with five (6%) confirmed to have EoE. Another study of children with recurrent croup found that 9% had EoE.[10] Kubik and coworkers[35] reported 13% (36 of 251) of patients confirmed with EoE based on biopsy criteria presented initially with airway complaints of stridor, dysphonia, repeated croup, and persistent cough. Yet another study found that 27% of patients with recurrent croup had EoE.[36]

KEY POINTS

- Work-up for patients with recurrent croup and/or persistent upper airway complaints should include examination of the esophagus for presence of EoE.

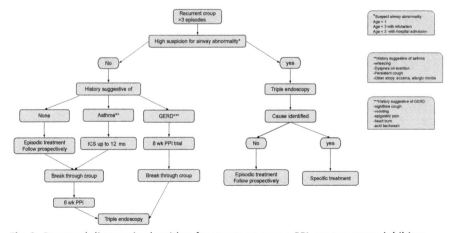

Fig. 2. Proposed diagnostic algorithm for recurrent croup. PPI, proton pump inhibitor.

EVALUATION AND MANAGEMENT OF RECURRENT CROUP

Acute croup can be frightening to parents and often prompts a visit to the emergency room. Recurrent croup episodes are often stressful for families and require repeated usage of steroids. A referral to a multidisciplinary aerodigestive team is recommended for the patient with recurrent or atypical croup. Evaluation by an aerodigestive team provides for consultation with pediatric subspecialists in otolaryngology, pulmonology, and gastroenterology and for the development of an integrated diagnostic and treatment plan (**Fig. 2**).

Patients with a high index of suspicion for major airway pathology, such as age less than 1, and age less than 3 with a history of intubation or hospital admission, should proceed directly to combined laryngoscopy, bronchoscopy, and esophagoscopy (triple endoscopy). Triple endoscopy entails detailed examination of the aerodigestive tract assessing for glottic, subglottic, and tracheal abnormalities; evidence for atopic airway disease; signs suggestive of GERD, and the presence of EoE. Bronchoalveolar lavage is used to assess for evidence of missed infection, microaspiration, and/or atopic markers. Despite identified risk factors for airway abnormality, review of the literature reports that only a small percentage of patients with recurrent croup had significant airway pathology that required surgical intervention. It is also reasonable to consider a trial of medical management before proceeding with triple endoscopy.

Although croup responds well to systemic steroids, even a short steroid burst (defined as <14 days) can lead to toxicity. Toxicity from systemic steroids occurs in a dose- and duration-dependent fashion but can occur even after a single burst of steroids.[37–39] Adverse effects tend to wane within 30 days of completing treatment; however, there is a potential for cumulative toxicity with repeated bursts of steroids. Because recurrent croup has a strong association with asthma, preventive therapy is extrapolated from treatment of asthma. Based on current asthma treatment guidelines, preventive inhaled corticosteroid (ICS) should be considered for patients who use two or more steroid bursts per year.[40] Because croup is an episodic illness, it is reasonable to use preventive ICS for at least a 12-month period to assess the efficacy for recurrent croup. If a patient has a history suggestive of GERD, or has a breakthrough episode of croup while on ICS, it is reasonable to consider treatment of gastroesophageal reflux with a proton pump inhibitor[41] course before proceeding to triple endoscopy.

Triple endoscopy should be performed on patients experiencing breakthrough episodes of croup after a reasonable trial of antiasthma and/or anti-GERD therapy, to rule out an underlying airway disorder and EoE. Identification of EoE on esophagoscopy should then prompt a referral to allergist for detailed allergy evaluation and gastroenterologist for medical care.

Using triple endoscopy with a multidisciplinary approach yields an underlying cause in up to 70% of cases.[11] Finding the cause for recurrent croup often relieves parental anxiety. Specific diagnoses provide the treatment team with the tools to fine tune therapy. Despite detailed work-up, no cause is found in approximately 30% of recurrent croup cases.[11] Patients without a clear cause or failed empirical therapy should continue to have close follow-up. Because of the potential for cumulative systemic steroid toxicity, high-dose nebulized budesonide is considered as an effective and safer alternative to multiple doses of systemic steroids to manage acute episodes of croup.[42–44]

KEY POINTS

- Consider referring patients with recurrent croup for work-up.

- Consider triple endoscopy in patients with strong suspicion for airway pathology.
- Consider antiasthma and anti-GERD treatment in patients without a strong suspicion for airway pathology.

CLINICS CARE POINTS

- Patients with recurrent croup that are less than 1 year of age or less than 3 years of age with history of intubation should have triple endoscopy performed to look for structural airway abnormalities.
- Patients without risk factor for airway abnormality should be screened for possible asthma and/or GERD and be treated empirically for asthma or GERD.
- Patients experiencing breakthrough croup on medical management should undergo triple endoscopy.
- Look for eosinophilic esophagitis in patients with recurrent croup unresponsive to antiasthma treatment, unresponsive to anti-GERD treatment, or with any signs of dysphagia.

DISCLOSURE

Nothing to disclose.

REFERENCES

1. Johnson DW. Croup. BMJ Clin Evid 2014;2014, 0321. Published 2014 Sep 29.David Wyatt.
2. Bjornson CL, Johnson DW. Croup Lancet 2008;371(9609):329–39.
3. Asher MI. Infections of the upper respiratory tract. Pediatric respiratory medicine. Mosby; 1999.
4. Uba A. Infraglottic and bronchial infections. Prim Care 1996;23(4):759–91.
5. Van Bever HP, Wieringa MH, Weyler JJ, et al. Croup and recurrent croup: their association with asthma and allergy. An epidemiological study on 5-8-year-old children. Eur J Pediatr 1999;158(3):253–7.
6. Chun R, Preciado DA, Zalzal GH, et al. Utility of bronchoscopy for recurrent croup. Ann Otol Rhinol Laryngol 2009;118(7):495–9.
7. Jabbour N, Parker NP, Finkelstein M, et al. Incidence of operative endoscopy findings in recurrent croup. Otolaryngol Head Neck Surg 2011;144(4):596–601.
8. Rankin I, Wang SM, Waters A, et al. The management of recurrent croup in children. J Laryngol Otol 2013;127(5):494–500.
9. Delany DR, Johnston DR. Role of direct laryngoscopy and bronchoscopy in recurrent croup. Otolaryngol Head Neck Surg 2015;152(1):159–64.
10. Hodnett BL, Simons JP, Riera KM, Mehta DK, Maguire RC. Objective endoscopic findings in patients with recurrent croup: 10-year retrospective analysis. Int J Pediatr Otorhinolaryngol 2015;79(12):2343–7.
11. Hiebert JC, Zhao YD, Willis EB. Bronchoscopy findings in recurrent croup: a systematic review and meta-analysis. Int J Pediatr Otorhinolaryngol 2016;90:86–90.
12. Duval M, Tarasidis G, Grimmer JF. Role of operative airway evaluation in children with recurrent croup: a retrospective cohort study. Clin Otolaryngol 2015;40:227–33.
13. Saraswatula A, McShane D, Tideswell D, et al. Mediastinal masses masquerading as common respiratory conditions of childhood: a case series. Eur J Pediatr 2009;168(11):1395–9.

14. Fraga JC, Jennings RW, Kim PC. Pediatric tracheomalacia. Semin Pediatr Surg 2016;25(3):156–64.
15. Coughran A, Balakrishnan K, Ma Y, et al. The relationship between croup and gastroesophageal reflux: a systematic review and meta-analysis. Laryngoscope 2021;131(1):209–17.
16. Halstead LA. Gastroesophageal reflux: a critical factor in pediatric subglottic stenosis. Otolaryngol Head Neck Surg 1999;120(5):683–8.
17. Halstead LA. Role of gastroesophageal reflux in pediatric upper airway disorders. Otolaryngol Head Neck Surg 1999;120(2):208–14.
18. Waki EY, Madgy N, Belenky WM. The incidence of gastroesophageal reflux in recurrent croup. International J Ped Otolaryngol 1995;32:223–32.
19. Duval M, Meier J, Asfour F, et al. Association between follicular tracheitis and gastroesophageal reflux. Int J Pediatr Otorhinolaryngol 2016;82:8–11.
20. Kwong K, Hoa M, Coticchia JM. Recurrent croup presentation, diagnosis, and management. Am J Otolaryngol 2007;28(6):401–7.
21. Hoa M, Kingsley EL, Coticchia JM. Correlating the clinical course of recurrent croup with endoscopic findings: a retrospective observational study. Ann Otol Rhinol Laryngol 2008;117(6):464–9.
22. Krishnan U, Paul S, Messina I, Soma M. Correlation between laryngobronchoscopy and pepsin in the diagnosis of extra-oesophageal reflux. J Laryngol Otol 2015;129(6):572–9.
23. Justiz Vaillant AA, Modi P, Jan A. Atopy. In: StatPearls. Treasure Island (FL): StatPearls Publishing; 2021.
24. O'Byrne PM, Inman MD. Airway hyperresponsiveness. Chest 2003;123(3 Suppl). 411S-6S.
25. Fahy JV, O'Byrne PM. Reactive airways disease". A lazy term of uncertain meaning that should be abandoned. Am J Respir Crit Care Med 2001;163(4):822–3.
26. GKjellman NI. Recurrent croup and allergy. Arch Dis Child 1981;56(11):893–4.
27. Hide DW. Guyer BM. Recurrent croup. Arch Dis Child 1985;60(6):585–6.
28. Zach M, Erben A, Olinsky A. Croup, recurrent group, allergy, and airways hyperreactivity. Arch Dis Child 1981;56(5):336–41.
29. Castro-Rodríguez JA, Holberg CJ, Morgan WJ, et al. Relation of two different subtypes of croup before age three to wheezing, atopy, and pulmonary function during childhood: a prospective study. Pediatrics 2001;107(3):512–8.
30. Kelly EA, Linn D, Keppel KL, Noel RJ, Chun RH. Otolaryngologic surgeries are frequent in children with eosinophilic esophagitis. Ann Otol Rhinol Laryngol 2015;124(5):355–60.
31. Dauer EH, Ponikau JU, Smyrk TC, Murray JA, Thompson DM. Airway manifestations of pediatric eosinophilic esophagitis: a clinical and histopathologic report of an emerging association. Ann Otol Rhinol Laryngol 2006;115(7):507–17.
32. Thompson DM, Arora AS, Romero Y, Dauer EH. Eosinophilic esophagitis: its role in aerodigestive tract disorders. Otolaryngol Clin North Am. 2006;39(1):205–21.
33. Otteson TD, Mantle BA, Casselbrant ML, Goyal A. The otolaryngologic manifestations in children with eosinophilic esophagitis. Int J Pediatr Otorhinolaryngol 2012;76(1):116–9.
34. Cooper T, Kuruvilla G, Persad R, El-Hakim H. Atypical croup: association with airway lesions, atopy, and esophagitis. Otolaryngol Head Neck Surg 2012; 147(2):209–14.
35. Kubik M, Thottam P, Shaffer A, Choi S. The role of the otolaryngologist in the evaluation and diagnosis of eosinophilic esophagitis. Laryngoscope 2017;127(6): 1459–64.

36. Greifer M, Santiago MT, Tsirilakis K, Cheng JC, Smith LP. Pediatric patients with chronic cough and recurrent croup: the case for a multidisciplinary approach. Int J Pediatr Otorhinolaryngol 2015;79(5):749–52.
37. Saag KG, Furst DE. Major side effects of systemic glucocorticoids. UpToDate 2021.
38. Yao TC, Wang JY, Chang SM, et al. Association of oral corticosteroid bursts with severe adverse events in children [published correction appears in JAMA Pediatr. 2021 Jul 1;175(7):751]. JAMA Pediatr 2021;175(7):723–9.
39. Yao TC, Huang YW, Chang SM, Tsai SY, Wu AC, Tsai HJ. Association between oral corticosteroid bursts and severe adverse events: a nationwide population-based cohort study. Ann Intern Med 2020;173(5):325–30.
40. Guidelines for the Diagnosis and Management of Asthma. National Asthma Education and Prevention Program. Expert Panel Report 3 (EPR-3. National Heart Lung Blood Institute, 2007.
41. Poddar U. Gastroesophageal reflux disease (GERD) in children. Paediatr Int Child Health 2019;39(1):7–12.
42. MFitzgerald D. Mellis C, Johnson M, Allen H, Cooper P, Van Asperen P. Nebulized budesonide is as effective as nebulized adrenaline in moderately severe croup. Pediatrics 1996;97(5):722–5.
43. OKlassen TP. Watters LK, Feldman ME, Sutcliffe T, Rowe PC. The efficacy of nebulized budesonide in dexamethasone-treated outpatients with croup. Pediatrics 1996;97(4):463–6.
44. PKlassen TP. Feldman ME, Watters LK, Sutcliffe T, Rowe PC. Nebulized budesonide for children with mild-to-moderate croup. N Engl J Med 1994;331(5):285–9.

Pediatric Voice

Scott M. Rickert, MD[a],*, Eadaoin O'Cathain, MD[b]

KEYWORDS

- Voice • Dysphonia • Pediatric • Hoarseness • Voice therapy • Speech

KEY POINTS

- Pediatric dysphonia is commonly underdiagnosed and may cause social isolation and impact a patient's academic, social, and emotional life.
- Subjective and objective measures can be used to best evaluate pediatric dysphonia in a combined visit to an otolaryngologist and a speech language pathologist. Typically, pediatric dysphonia is best managed with an experienced multidisciplinary team.
- Stroboscopy is a useful objective tool to identify causes of pediatric dysphonia and can evaluate motion as well as mucosal pathologic condition.
- Treatment of pediatric dysphonia can vary greatly and depends on the nature of the dysphonia. Treatment includes conservative treatment of observation, voice therapy, medical therapy and interventional treatment of injection medialization, surgical intervention, and laryngeal reinnervation.
- General management of the pediatric airway is a balance of maintaining a good airway while maintaining a good voice. Optimizing airway and voice remains the quintessential challenge in the management of pediatric dysphonia.

INTRODUCTION

Voice disorders in the pediatric population are as varied as they are in the adult population. There is a wide spectrum of "normal" voice in the pediatric population, which varies by age, sex, and pubertal development. It is important to note that different adults (parents, teachers, speech language pathologists, pediatricians) interacting with the child may perceive the child's voice differently. These opinions may not be in agreement as to the whether the child is dysphonic nor the degree of dysphonia the child may have. This range of opinion provides a complicating factor in discerning the presence of a voice disorder and how to manage it appropriately. It is estimated that dysphonia will affect between 4% and 23% of children at some stage in their development.[1] In contrast to their adult counterparts, children with dysphonia are likely to have a self-limiting benign cause. The widespread, simplistic view of the

[a] Pediatric Otolaryngology, NYU Langone Health, 240 East 38th Street, 14th Floor, New York, NY 10016, USA; [b] Cochlear Implant and Complex Otology, Salford Royal Foundation Trust, Manchester, UK
* Corresponding author.
E-mail address: scott.rickert@nyulangone.org

Pediatr Clin N Am 69 (2022) 329–347
https://doi.org/10.1016/j.pcl.2022.01.003
0031-3955/22/© 2022 Elsevier Inc. All rights reserved.

pediatric hoarse voice as something to outgrow without treatment nor follow-up can be a great disservice to the patients and their families. The most common causes of dysphonia in children are due to vocal misuse, benign lesions, and infectious causes, including human papillomavirus (HPV) causing papillomatosis. Most of these causes will improve with input from speech language pathologists and by taking a watch-and-wait approach. It is often the case that as a child grows, and the vocal fold lengthens, and its dynamics change. With time, growth, and changes in puberty, these dysphonic issues can resolve. It has been reported that children with dysphonia can sometimes be unaware of their condition, which can cause problems when trying to motivate these children to complete treatment. It has also been shown that children with dysphonia can sometimes be judged more negatively than children with no voice disorders.[2]

It is therefore crucial to take a history from the patient's caregivers, including their teachers, as the reporting and assessment of severity of dysphonia has been shown to vary widely from patient to caregiver. It is also prudent to take a comprehensive history from the patient themselves, where appropriate. Sometimes there can be underlying anxieties and stressors that may precipitate or exacerbate dysphonia, for which the patient may need additional treatment and support. It is also important to understand that dysphonia in a child may cause social isolation and reduced involvement in school and sporting activities. It helps to be aware of the potential impact that dysphonia can have on a patient's academic, social, and emotional life.

Significant advances in pediatric voice over the past decade in evaluation, diagnosis, and management of pediatric voice disorders have improved both short-term and long-term outcomes for the dysphonic child.

Practitioners should have a thorough understanding of anatomy and physiology, how to accurately work up a pediatric voice disorder, and how to efficiently treat voice disorders.

ANATOMY AND PHYSIOLOGY

The larynx grows and develops significantly from birth to adulthood. In the neonate, the larynx sits at the level of C3-C4. By around the age of 15 years, the larynx sits at the level of C6-C7. In a neonate, simultaneous feeding and respiration are possible. In older children, the vocal fold consists of 3 layers. From deep to superficial, these consist of the vocalis muscle, the lamina propria (which consists of 3 layers: deep, intermediate, and superficial), and the epithelium. Newborn vocal cords differ from those of an older child or adult, in that the lamina propria consists of only 1 layer of loose collagen fibers between the vocalis muscle and the epithelium.[3] As children grow, their vocal folds also lengthen. It has been proven that there is no difference between male and female vocal cords in early childhood. However, this changes during puberty, when male vocal cords lengthen, and their larynx grows more dramatically than in female adolescents.[4]

The superior and recurrent laryngeal branches of the vagus nerve (cranial nerve X) innervate the laryngopharynx. The vocal cords are innervated by the recurrent laryngeal nerves. These branch from the vagus nerves in the upper thorax and reenter the neck from the thoracic inlet. They travel in the tracheoesophageal groove superiorly to their entrance in the larynx. The right recurrent laryngeal nerve travels under the right subclavian artery, and the left recurrent laryngeal nerve loops under the aortic arch. It is important to remember that mediastinal pathologic condition or cardiac surgery in a baby can be a cause of iatrogenic vocal cord palsy. The superior laryngeal nerve travels along the pharynx and separates into the internal and external branches.

These supply sensory innervation to the supraglottis and motor innervation to the cricothyroid muscle. The rest of the larynx is supplied by the recurrent laryngeal nerve for motor and sensory innervation.

Phonation occurs when exhaled air from the lungs passes between the vocal cords and causes oscillation of the mucosa of the vocal folds relative to the thyroarytenoid muscles and vocal ligaments. The intrinsic laryngeal muscles adjust the tension and position of the vocal folds, which creates changes in pitch and frequency of the voice. Contraction of the thyroarytenoid and cricothyroid muscles shorten and lengthen the vocal folds, respectively, creating lower and higher pitches of voice. Articulation is created through fine control of the tongue and lips. Resonance is created in the airway above the level of the vocal cords. The size of the pharynx, oral and nasal cavities, and larynx change with age and create changes in resonance, particularly in boys. Loudness of voice is dependent on the level of subglottic pressure involved during speech.

ASSESSMENT

A full history should include birth history, and any history of birth trauma, any history of prematurity or intubation, history of tracheostomy placement, previous cardiac or mediastinal surgery, history of reflux, history of asthma or other chronic airway disease should be elicited. It is important to be aware that a child with chronic dysphonia may be deemed by their parents to have a normal voice. Therefore, referrals to otolaryngology may come from colleagues in speech language pathology initially.

On examination, general inspection should include assessment of ease of respiration and presence of stridor. A head and neck examination should rule out any evidence of craniofacial abnormalities or any syndromic features. A nasal and throat examination should also be performed to assess for nasal obstruction, adenotonsillar hypertrophy, or palatal insufficiency. The quality of the child's voice should be noted, to include any sign of a weak or breathy voice, coarseness, whisper, or strained voice. Resonance is usually described as either normal, hypernasal, or hyponasal. There might be evidence of a variation in pitch, restricted range, decreased voice projection, voice breaks, or abnormal resonance.

Popular tools for self or parental assessment of voice include the CAPE-V questionnaire (Consensus Auditory-Perceptual Evaluation of Voice) and the Pediatric Voice Handicap Index (pVHI) (**Fig. 1**).[5] The PVRQOL (Pediatric Voice Related Quality of Life) and PVOS (Pediatric Voice Outcome Survey) are other useful questionnaires.[6] It should be noted that some of these tools will require parental assessment of the child's quality of life and so may not be entirely accurate. These tools can be used at initial assessment and also following intervention, to determine whether the intervention has helped. All of these children should be seen by a team of professionals who are experienced in the management of pediatric dysphonia. These teams generally consist of a pediatric otolaryngologist in conjunction with a speech language pathologist, who performs aerodynamic and acoustic evaluation. The speech language pathologists also assess the child's voice subjectively and objectively. Objective measures include assessment of pitch, range, loudness, shimmer, and jitter. These children will often have audiometric testing to ensure there is no element of hearing loss contributing to possible vocal misuse. When there is any concern for concomitant symptoms, such as cough, throat clearing, or weakness, that may be affecting the voice, these children will also be assessed by a pediatric pulmonologist, a pediatric allergist, pediatric gastroenterologist, or pediatric neurologist along with the speech language pathologist.

Subject Number: _____   Date: _____

I would rate my/my child's talkativeness as the following (circle response) | To be filled out by Staff:

1	2	3	4	5	6	7
Quiet Listener			Average Talker			Extremely Talkative

F= _____
P= _____
E= _____
Total= _____

Talkativeness: _____

Instructions: These are statements that many people have used to describe their voices and the effects of their voices on their lives. Circle the response that indicates how frequently you have the same experience.

0 = Never   1 = Almost Never   2 = Sometimes   3 = Almost always   4 = Always

Part I - F

1) My child's voice makes it difficult for people to hear him/her.   0 1 2 3 4

2) People have difficulty understanding my child in a noisy room.   0 1 2 3 4

3) At home, we have difficulty hearing my child when he/she calls through the house.   0 1 2 3 4

4) My child tends to avoid communicating because of his/her voice.   0 1 2 3 4

5) My child speaks with friends, neighbors, or relatives less often because of his/her voice.   0 1 2 3 4

6) People ask my child to repeat him/herself when speaking face to face.   0 1 2 3 4

7) My child's voice difficulties restrict personal, educational, and social activities.   0 1 2 3 4

Part II - P

1) My child runs out of air when talking.   0 1 2 3 4

2) The sound of my child's voice changes throughout the day.   0 1 2 3 4

3) People ask, "What's wrong with your child's voice?".   0 1 2 3 4

4) My child's voice sounds dry, raspy, and/or hoarse.   0 1 2 3 4

5) The quality of my child's voice is unpredictable.   0 1 2 3 4

6) My child uses a great deal of effort to speak.   0 1 2 3 4

7) My child's voice is worse in the evening.   0 1 2 3 4

0 = Never   1 = Almost Never   2 = Sometimes   3 = Almost always   4 = Always

Fig. 1. Pediatric voice handicap index.

INITIAL DIAGNOSTIC WORKUP

The initial investigation after voice assessment for any child with dysphonia is a flexible nasoendoscopy. This can be done in the clinic or by the bedside in the acute setting. Topical lidocaine without epinephrine in combination with a nasal decongestant can be applied to the anterior nasal cavities via cottonoids or via spray application to provide some topical relief during the examination. In younger children, a caregiver will need to have the child seated on their lap, with both people facing the endoscopist. A tower plus camera attachment to the scope should be used for recording the scope and to aid in facilitating a safe distance between the ENT surgeon and the patient and caregiver. The smallest diameter of a flexible nasoendoscope suggested for pediatric use is 2.1 mm. Typically, the small-caliber scopes are more comfortable to the patient on examination. It is also important to note that the larger the diameter of the scope, the better quality the associated image, so it is an important balance to limit discomfort while not sacrificing image quality and limiting diagnostic abilities.

Stroboscopy should also be performed in any patient with a concern for a voice disorder. This aids not only in assessing gross movement of the larynx and movement of the arytenoids but also in assessing the microstructure of the vocal fold and elucidate any evidence of lesion or scarring. In particular, it aids in the assessment of vocal cord symmetry, the mucosal wave, and glottis closure. Stroboscopy can be performed with either a rigid or flexible scope. The advantages of using the rigid strobe are that the image quality is excellent and that it has a zoom function. Disadvantages include possible discomfort while holding the mouth open, and potential damage to the teeth if a patient bites or is noncompliant. It is also possible to use a flexible strobe scope, which is passed in the usual transnasal approach, thereby being more readily tolerated for younger children.

A child-sized rigid strobe can be purchased, which is of a smaller diameter than an adult strobe. To use this, a child must be very compliant; therefore, it is more useful in older children or adolescents, although mature children as young as 3 to 4 years of age can tolerate a rigid examination well. The tongue is protruded and held with a gauze swab. Antifog solution is placed on the tip of the scope. When the patient opens their mouth, the rigid scope is passed through the mouth to sit over the larynx. It is often possible to use the intraoral rigid scope in a child without local anesthesia, as their larynx is more superiorly situated than in an adult. If a flexible stroboscopy approach is used, the flexible stroboscopes are slightly larger than the smallest flexible nasoendoscopes at 3.1 mm but are well tolerated even on younger children. This method is more easily tolerated, with no age restrictions. Topical anesthetic to nose becomes an essential part of a successful flexible examination.

A microphone is used to help sync the audio to the image in both rigid and flexible stroboscopy. Stroboscopy uses flashes of light, which synchronize at a slightly slower speed to the vocal fold vibration, which is picked up by the microphone. This allows vocal fold vibration to be appreciated in what appears to be slow motion. The mucosal wave, symmetry, and glottic closure can all be appreciated in greater detail using stroboscopy. A visualized setup of the needed equipment is shown in **Fig. 2**.

Different sounds on vocalization should be performed to assess the voice. Sniffing causes abduction of the vocal cords, which allows assessment of the movement of the cords and arytenoids. In an older child, the recitation of a paragraph will allow for more in-depth analysis of the quality of the voice.

Laryngeal ultrasound (**Fig. 3**) is a newer technique for evaluating the anatomy and movement of the larynx. It can be a helpful diagnostic tool where a child is fearful of nasendoscopy or an examination is particularly difficult to obtain anatomically. It can be particularly useful when evaluating for a laryngeal cyst or distinguishing vocal cord palsy, as patients are much more compliant with the ultrasound examination. It will not obtain information on the mucosal wave itself but is very useful to assess asymmetries in motion or in anatomy.

In some situations, it may be necessary to further assess the airway under anesthesia. This provides a microscopic viewpoint under direct visualization and the ability to palpate and examine any areas of concern. In these cases, one can perform a direct microlaryngoscopy as part of a broader endoscopic airway evaluation. One can also potentially include a flexible bronchoscopy with the same anesthetic to assess the airway below the level of the glottis, to rule out any other dynamic tracheal or bronchial anomaly.

In the case of a unilateral or bilateral vocal cord paralysis, it is important to perform imaging to rule out any underlying cause. As an example, an MRI brain scan can be helpful to rule out an Arnold-Chiari malformation, which could cause a bilateral vagal nerve palsy. Imaging of the neck and thorax is also important to rule out any pathologic condition along the course of the recurrent laryngeal nerve or nerves. In general, MRI is preferable to computed tomography (CT), as it does not involve a radiation dose. It is worth noting that children older than a few months of age will likely need either sedation or a general anesthetic to tolerate MRI or CT scanning. Dynamic voice CT (**Fig. 4**) is a newer investigation that is used in some children with previous history of multiple complex airway surgeries.

In children with a history of esophageal reflux, or evidence of chronic laryngitis, erythema, or edema of the arytenoids, a contrast swallow study or esophagoscopy can be performed to assess localized inflammation that may affect voice. They may also

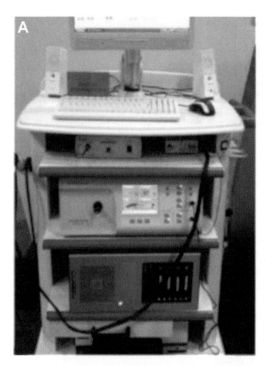
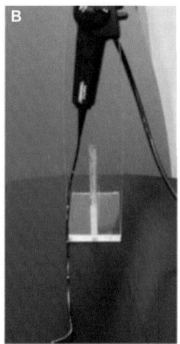
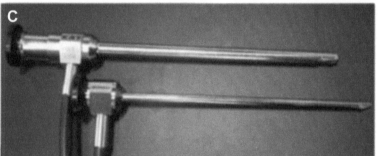

Fig. 2. *A)* Stack system used. (*B*) Flexiscope with chip-in-tip for stroboscopy. (*C*) Rigid stoboscopy scopes. (*Adapted from Recent Advances in Otolaryngology-Head and Neck Surgery. Publisher: Jaypee, 2012. Anil K Lalwani, Markus H F Pfister, page 170.*)

require assessment by a gastroenterologist and a clinical assessment of swallow performed by a speech language pathologist if there is concern.

Laryngeal electromyography (EMG) is helpful to assess vocal cord paresis versus paralysis. In adults and older children, one can perform this in the clinic setting with mild discomfort to the patient. In younger children, an awake laryngeal EMG is typically not tolerated, and it is usually performed under a general anesthesia and with the aid of an electrophysiology physician. The data obtained under a general anesthesia may not be as diagnostically distinct as an awake laryngeal EMG without anesthesia but can help assess and compare laterality in the cases of concern for vocal fold paresis/immobility. One can also perform a diagnostic microlaryngoscopy examination under anesthesia at the same time as the laryngeal EMG to distinguish vocal fold immobility from neurogenic paresis.

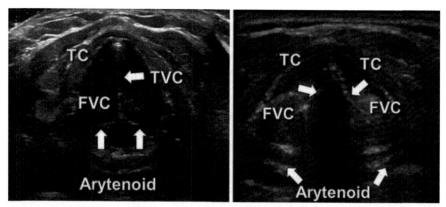

Fig. 3. Laryngeal ultrasound. TC, thyroid cartilage; TVC, true vocal cord; FVC, false vocal cord. Arrows point to the anatomic structures. (Carneiro-Pla D. (2017) *Transcutaneous Laryngeal Ultrasonography: Technical Performance and Interpretation. In: Milas M., Mandel S., Langer J. (eds) Advanced Thyroid and Parathyroid Ultrasound. Springer, Cham. https://doi. org/10.1007/978-3-319-44100-9_32)*

DIFFERENTIAL DIAGNOSIS AND TREATMENT
Common Causes of Pediatric Dysphonia

Laryngopharyngeal reflux

Laryngitis, inflammation of the larynx, can be caused by laryngopharyngeal reflux (LPR). Symptoms can include globus pharyngeus and chronic cough or throat-clearing. Signs on flexible scope can include edema, erythema, and pachydermia. Diagnosis of LPR requires some thought, as symptoms of throat clearing or cough may be arising from other causes as well. General suspicion of LPR should have

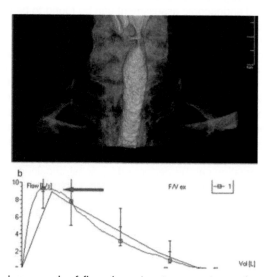

Fig. 4. F/V, flow volume graph of flow dynamics. *Arrows* point to the concerning area of narrowed airway. Ruane, Laurence, and Lau, Kenneth and Low, Kathy and Crossett, Marcus and Vallance, Neil and Bardin, Philip (2014). (*From Dynamic 320-slice CT larynx for detection and management of idiopathic bilateral vocal cord paralysis. Respirology Case Reports. 2. 10.1002/rcr2.37.*)

follow-up with a gastroenterologist, and treatment includes proton-pump inhibitors and lifestyle modifications, including weight loss. As with all medications in children, care should be taken to prescribe reflux medications based on age and weight. A referral to gastroenterology is essential in recalcitrant cases for further workup, including esophagogastroduodenoscopy (EGD) or impedance probe.

Vocal fold movement impairment

This is the second most common congenital laryngeal anomaly after laryngomalacia. It usually presents between birth and 2 months of age. It can be symptomatic of a multi-system anomaly involving the central nervous system and cardiopulmonary anomalies. Vocal fold movement impairment (VFMI) can be further associated with laryngeal clefts or subglottic stenosis. Unilateral VFMI is more common than bilateral, and left unilateral VFMI is more common than right VFMI. Unilateral VFMI can present as a weak or breathy cry, whereas bilateral VMFI may present with respiratory distress and stridor with a surprisingly normal voice. Diagnosis of VMFI can be done through a thorough history and physical examination. History of thoracic surgery should yield suspicion of VFMI. Intubation is an exceeding rare cause of VFMI.[7] Endoscopic assessment of the vocal fold (through flexible or rigid stroboscopy) is essential to understanding the laterality of any movement impairment and degree of impairment. Laryngeal ultrasound is becoming a good noninvasive diagnostic tool to diagnose VFMI. Imaging of the laryngeal nerve pathway is an essential part of the diagnostic workup from the base of skull to the chest to rule out concerning lesions.

In unilateral VFMI, sometimes it will resolve with time. Observation is appropriate in cases whereby there is no known cause and no evidence of respiratory distress or difficulty feeding. In cases of vocal cord palsy caused by cardiac surgery, it has been shown that around 5% of babies or children undergoing surgeries of the aortic arch can be left with a left-sided vocal cord palsy.[8] Therefore, it is important to screen these children before discharge and to have a high index of suspicion in terms of diagnosis. Laryngeal EMG and endoscopic assessment can be found to be useful for assessing qualitative function of a vocal fold palsy and distinguish vocal fold immobility from neurogenic palsy.

In cases of nonresolving unilateral vocal cord palsy, medialization thyroplasty with injection or permanent implants, such as Gore-Tex or silicone, may be helpful. In adults, type I thyroplasty is performed usually under light sedation to confirm the quality of phonation with the implant in place, so that adjustments can be made. However, in children, they need a full general anesthetic, which can make placement of the graft somewhat challenging. It is worth mentioning that a younger child will outgrow the graft and so may require revision surgery if there is ongoing atrophy of the vocal fold. Therefore, it may be prudent to postpone thyroplasty surgery until they are older.

Laryngeal reinnervation can be performed by anastomosing the ansa cervicalis to the recurrent laryngeal nerve on the affected side. Laryngeal reinnervation has been proven to be beneficial in adults with chronic unilateral vocal cord paralysis. There are fewer studies in children. A review by Zur and colleagues[9] in 2015 showed that the largest benefit from reinnervation surgery was seen in children from 1 to 2 years after the initial vocal cord palsy, in cases of unknown cause. The advantages of reinnervation surgery include 1 procedure under general anesthesia that is low risk and does not preclude the use of medialization thyroplasty in the future. Disadvantages include no long-term data, the need for an incision in the neck, and the need to wait months for an outcome. Preoperative workup includes a full voice evaluation as detailed previously. It is important to discuss potential outcomes and set reasonable expectations with parents before surgery, including the need to wait many months, it is

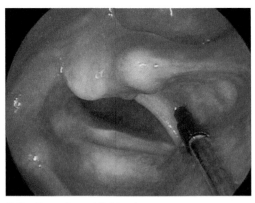

Fig. 5. Injection medialization of vocal fold palsy.

hoped, before having a successful improvement in voice quality. Laryngeal EMG may be helpful as an adjunct to diagnosis and planning; however, it may require a general anesthetic in a child. It is important to explain to the parents that after the surgery, the vocal cord may remain paralyzed, but the tone will be improved, hence resulting in a better closure of the cords and improved acoustics.

Temporary laryngeal injection just lateral to the vocal fold (**Fig. 5**) might be used before more permanent techniques, to test the possible outcomes if permanent surgery were to be performed. None of the current synthetic materials are permanent. Younger children undergoing injection medialization should stay overnight for pulse oximetry and observation to ensure no airway compromise following the procedure. If successful, vocal cord injection can be repeated, or more permanent surgery can be performed. Although there are no long-term studies to prove the benefits of early vocal cord injection following palsy, they have been shown in adults. Injectable materials include Gelfoam (6 weeks), Restalyne (3–6 months), and Cymetra (3–9 months). Longer-term options include Radiesse/Prolaryn (1–2 years) or fat (1–2 years or permanent). Choice of material used is influenced by the length of time desired for benefits to last, the risk/benefit profile of the material, and availability including cost.

Bilateral VFMI (**Fig. 6**) is much less common and can be a much more acute clinical situation. Typically, patients present with impaired breathing and stridor with a more normal voice when voicing. Swallowing issues may arise as well. Frequently, a swallow study is performed if there is any concern for dysphagia. If there is concern for a neurologic cause of bilateral VFMI, an MRI scan of the brain can be helpful to rule out an Arnold-Chiari malformation, which could cause a bilateral vagal nerve palsy in addition to the typical imaging workup of a vocal fold palsy.

Interventions for bilateral VFMI are designed to improve airflow and prevent airway compromise. Any intervention to provide a larger airway by definition decreases the ease of closure and can affect the voice. Interventions include both destructive and expansive techniques to provide a larger airway. Destructive techniques include scar release, vocal fold lateralization, vocal fold cordotomy, and arytenoidectomy. Expansive techniques include posterior cricoid graft placement. Other treatment options include reinnervation of the posterior cricoarytenoid muscle to provide neural input to a neurologically impaired vocal fold.

Laryngeal webs
Laryngeal webs (**Fig. 7**) may be congenital or acquired and typically affect the anterior margin of the vocal fold. In tethering a portion of the vocal folds together, the vibration

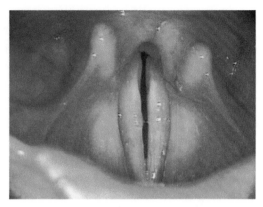

Fig. 6. Bilateral vocal fold paresis seen with rigid stroboscopy.

of the true margin of the vocal fold is altered and prevents a normal propagation of a mucosal wave. Repeated microlaryngoscopy with intervention is the most common cause of acquired laryngeal webs, which tend to be thinner than congenital webs. Congenital airway webs, 75% which are glottic in location, are formed because of a failure in recanalization of the glottis during development. A narrowed cricoid is associated with congenital glottic webs.

Velocardiofacial syndrome, a genetic deletion of 22q, is frequently associated with congenital webs. Therefore, all congenital webs should have a genetic workup in their treatment plan.[10] Laryngeal webs are notoriously difficult to treat, as the goal is to restore a normal vibrating vocal fold with proper propagation of the mucosal wave. Typically, cold sharp dissection is used in an endoscopic fashion, with or without placement of a keel to try and prevent reformation of the glottis web. If the cricoid is severely narrowed, an anterior cricoid split (endoscopic or open) or an anterior laryngotracheoplasty may be indicated in addition to prevent further reformation of the glottic web.

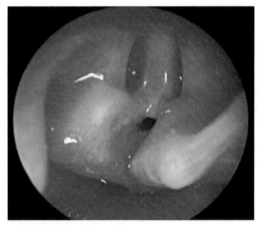

Fig. 7. Near complete congenital glottic web.

Benign Vocal Fold Lesions

Benign vocal fold lesions are the most common cause of dysphonia in children. The lesions can be congenital or acquired. Based on the location and nature of the lesion, conservative treatment can be effective. More aggressive interventions, such as microlaryngoscopy and removal of the lesion, are reserved for recalcitrant lesions that are adversely affecting voice and impacting the child's quality of life on a daily basis. Many children with mild dysphonia in the setting of a benign vocal fold lesion may continue to be treated conservatively as long as daily activities and daily interactions are not adversely affected.

Vocal fold nodules

These are the most common lesions causing dysphonia in children. They are caused by vocal misuse and abuse. They are bilateral and are found at the junction between the first one-third of the vocal fold and the subsequent two-thirds of the vocal fold. The vocal fold closure is described as an hourglass closure configuration. On stroboscopy, there can be a normal mucosal wave, or minimal changes of the mucosal wave. In general, vocal fold nodules respond very well to voice therapy and conservative treatment.

Vocal fold cysts

Vocal fold cysts are more often unilateral than bilateral, typically with a contralateral reactive lesion (**Fig. 8**). The location of a vocal fold cyst will determine the impact on the voice impact. These are distinguished from vocal fold nodules by videostroboscopy, as they impair the mucosal wave, depending on its size and location. These respond less predictably to voice therapy and often require surgery when adversely affecting voice and daily activities. Removal of a vocal fold cyst is routinely performed using the microflap technique under an outpatient anesthetic.

Vocal fold polyp

Polyps are an uncommon finding in children and much more commonly found in adults. They generally present unilaterally as a polypoid lesion from a typical submucosal bleeding episode. There can frequently be an associated contact lesion on the ipsilateral fold because of recurrent point contact from the polyp on the contralateral fold. They are treated conservatively initially, with voice therapy. Surgery with minimal disruption to the underlying cord is kept in reserve for recalcitrant polyps.

Vocal cord granuloma

Vocal cord granuloma can be associated with chronic cough or LPR inflaming the vocal fold mucosa (**Fig. 9**). Occasionally, they can occur as a result of previous intubation. These granulomas typically arise in the posterior third of the cord and present a few weeks after extubation. They can be treated conservatively with vocal rest and reflux medication and typically resolve with time. If they are large, impacting breathing, and causing stridor or do not respond to conservative treatment, they can be excised with an outpatient surgery.

Recurrent respiratory papillomatosis

Recurrent respiratory papillomatosis (RRP) is the second most common cause of dysphonia in children (**Figs. 10** and **11**). It is caused by HPV subtypes 6 and 11. Surgical debridement is the mainstay of treatment. Surgical debridement is most commonly performed using a cold technique of a microdebrider or other instrumentation as part of a microlaryngoscopy setup or with laser-aided surgery. During the initial surgery, a biopsy should always be taken to confirm the diagnosis. The primary goals of surgery are to reduce tumor burden, to decrease the chance of distal spread of

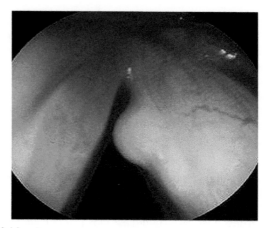

Fig. 8. Left vocal fold cyst.

disease, and to create a safe airway. It is also performed to improve voice quality, and it is hoped, to increase the time between surgeries. However, surgery is not curative. Most cases of RRP regress and "burn out" as the child grows and their immune system matures. Some adjuncts to surgery are KTP LASER (532n), Bevacizumab, and Cidofovir.[11] Bevacizumab is a recombinant antibody designed to bind vascular endothelial growth factor-A (VEGF-A) and inhibit VEGF receptor interaction. It is used as an intralesional adjunct in the management of RRP, although its use is off-label. Although no randomized control trials have occurred to date, results have been promising, with few side effects.[11] Cidofovir is a cytosine nucleotide analogue that inhibits the replication of DNA viruses by blocking viral DNA polymerase function. The mechanism of action in HPV and RRP is unclear; however, it is thought that it induces apoptosis and enhances the immune system. It is injected into the base of the papillomata once they have been debrided. Although it is well tolerated and has been found to be of benefit at certain doses, there is a theoretic risk of malignant transformation.[11]

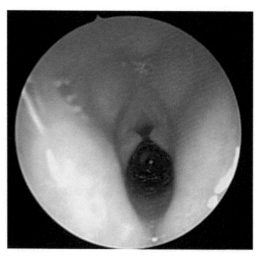

Fig. 9. Bilateral postintubation granulomas seen within conventional flexible laryngoscopy.

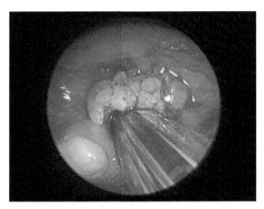

Fig. 10. Obstructive papilloma of the larynx.

Therefore, the parents of a child undergoing potential Cidofovir injection should be well counseled and provided with ample evidence before consenting to the treatment.

Quadrivalent HPV recombinant vaccine is frequently used when systemic treatment is deemed necessary. Systemic treatment is usually considered in cases of aggressive disease requiring more than 4 surgeries per year, or in cases of spread of disease in the distal airways, or rapid regrowth and airway compromise. A recent prospective study by Matsuzaki and colleagues[12] has shown significant reduction of RRP lesions in adults injected with the quadrivalent vaccine during their treatment. Intravenous therapies, such as Bevacizumab and interferon, can be considered in cases requiring more than 4 procedures per year; however, these are not instituted on a regular basis, as shown in a recent International Pediatric Otolaryngology Group consensus paper.[11] With better access to the vaccine for children, it is hoped there will ultimately be a reduction in the incidence of RRP.

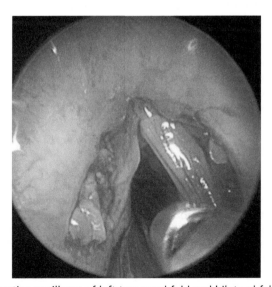

Fig. 11. Nonobstructive papilloma of left true vocal fold and bilateral false vocal folds.

Functional Voice Disorders

Functional disorders are caused by dysregulated laryngeal function. Up to 40% of adult patients have functional voice disorders,[13] whereas only 7% of children had a functional cause.[14] Functional disorders affecting the voice include muscle tension dysphonia, psychogenic dysphonia, and puberphonia. This causes a strained voice with pitch changes and occasional periods of aphonia. Treatment in these cases is often behavior modification in tandem with speech therapy. Occasionally, Botox can be considered in specific cases when conservative treatment has not been helpful.

Paradoxic vocal fold dysfunction

This is also called paradoxic vocal cord movement, laryngospasm, and exercise-induced laryngeal obstruction. A typical patient is a high achiever in school and an athlete This more commonly diagnosed in female patients than in male patients. Frequently, these patients have a history of asthma or exercise-induced asthma as well. They may also have a history of a psychological stressor or event that preceded or coincided with the onset of symptoms. Their symptoms of shortness of breath during paradoxic vocal fold movement classically do not improve with an inhaler. Episodes occur when the vocal cords adduct during inspiration, which causes stridor and a described "air hunger" and understandably associated anxiety. Future episodes can occur with minimal stimulation, and sometimes even without exercise. Pulmonary function tests can be performed, which may show a flattened inspiratory loop, or might be normal. Pediatric pulmonologists', otolaryngologists', and speech language pathologists' involvement are needed for best care. During an evaluation in the voice clinic, all routine investigations may appear normal. Treatment is often centered on the fact that it helps to diagnose the condition and acknowledge it. Breathing exercises with speech, and abdominal breathing with open throat breathing, can be taught to break episodes when they occur. These skills can be taught with biofeedback, for example, on a treadmill during flexible endoscopy. It can be useful to enlist the help of a psychologist/sports psychologist in managing these patients. In recalcitrant cases, a psychiatry evaluation can be considered, as can acupuncture, or exercise stress laryngoscopy (ESL). ESL is a laryngeal evaluation during exercise, which attempts to re-create the physiologic conditions experienced during episodes of this condition. The equipment needed to perform these investigations include a treadmill, a flexible scope or stroboscopy, a camera and tower, pulse oximetry, electrocardiogram, spirometry, and concurrent measurement of vital signs. It is important to thoroughly explain the procedure and demonstrate all of the equipment before beginning the investigation.

Puberphonia

Puberphonia is a disorder that occurs when there is a failure of the voice to alter from a higher pitch associated with early childhood to the lower vocal pitch of adolescence and adulthood. It may be due to a maladaptation to the psychological changes that occur during puberty. Hyperfunction of the cricothyroid muscle and muscular incoordination combined with the psychological uncertainties of puberty may be contributing factors. Children with this condition often have breathiness and decreased power of vocal projection. Treatment involves voice therapy and problem-directed psychotherapy.

Dysphonia in professional voice users

There is a particular subset of professional voice users who are children and face challenges with dysphonia in tandem with their adult counterparts because of their particular need for high-performance voice use. This is a type of functional disorder that benefits from a multidisciplinary team approach by otolaryngologist, a voice therapist, voice coach, and occasionally with a psychologist to best serve the demanding voice needs of these professional performers.

Less Common Causes of Pediatric Dysphonia

Dysphonia following airway surgery and airway reconstruction surgery

Laryngotracheal stenosis and reconstruction surgery can adversely affect the voice. Premature births are on the increase in many countries.[15] As more babies are surviving premature births and requiring tracheostomies in their first few months of life,[16] it is important to recognize the potential impact of laryngotracheal reconstruction surgeries on voice. During these surgeries, the primary goal is improvement of and creation of a safe airway without a tracheotomy tube. Voice concerns are generally of secondary importance to airway concerns. These patients may have had multiple surgeries in the past, potentially creating scarring, bowing, or height mismatch of the vocal folds not allowing a consistent mucosal wave along the entire vocal fold yielding a dysphonic voice (**Fig. 12**). If the posterior glottis is too wide after reconstruction, there can be the creation of a posterior glottic gap and inability to fully close the glottis effectively. This results in a supraglottic speech pattern and dysphonia secondary to it. Following these surgeries and decannulation of tracheostomies, these children will frequently go on to have concerns around socializing, sports participation, and ultimately potential voice concerns affecting choice of occupation. One innovative way of assessing movement of the larynx in these patients is to perform a dynamic CT voice, which may help in diagnosing anatomic areas in need of further surgery or speech therapy. In these patients, the goal of voice "restoration" involves changing to glottic from supraglottic voice and improving loudness. Vocal fold injection may help to test for benefit of further surgery and may help glottic insufficiencies. However, it will not improve a posterior glottic gap. For posterior glottic gap after laryngotracheal reconstruction, an endoscopic posterior cricoid reduction in an older child has been shown to reduce a posterior glottic gap.[17] This can be performed with a laser. Candidacy for this procedure is decided with voice evaluation in the clinic, followed by dynamic voice CT and a screening laryngoscopy and endoscopy.

Dysphonia in children with craniofacial anomalies

Children with craniofacial anomalies often develop dysphonia. In 1 study, 10% of these patients who were evaluated for dysphonia were found to have an organic vocal fold pathologic condition causing their symptoms.[18,19] Half of these findings were attributable to iatrogenic causes. Issues with resonance caused by hypernasality and hyponasality were also common. The pVHI score was found to be a helpful adjunct in diagnosing those children who would benefit from speech and voice therapy as an initial treatment.

Controversies in Management of Vocal Fold Pathologic Conditions

One of the biggest controversies in pediatric dysphonia is when is it appropriate to operate on children with vocal fold pathologic conditions. There are no clear guidelines. However, most practitioners think that after the age of 7 years recalcitrant benign lesions may require surgery. Of course, most practitioners adopt a conservative approach for as long as possible. It is sensible to consider the maturity of a child

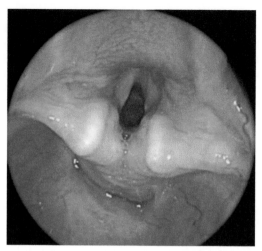

Fig. 12. Post-reconstruction dysphonia with height mismatch of vocal folds.

before suggesting surgery, as all postoperative patients will need to commit to a voice therapy program as part of the rehabilitation process. If the child is not considered mature enough to partake in a preoperative voice therapy program, then surgery should be postponed until they are ready to engage with a speech language pathologist.

There is no definitive decision on how much voice therapy is needed in most cases. It is reasonable to undergo a trial of 10 sessions or up to 2 months of voice therapy at the least, before reassessment and decision regarding further/different therapies or management strategies. Treatment of underlying LPR, gastroesophageal reflux disease(GERD), or eosinophilic esophagitis is essential. When conservative management fails, it is pertinent to consider changing the type of voice therapy, or entertaining the possibility of unilateral vocal fold surgery if necessary initially, and choosing to operate based on the patient's and family's perceptions and opinions. It is important to stress to the patient and family that there is an expected voice rest period required following surgery. If this is not deemed possible, then surgery may not be a wise choice, and conservative treatment may be a wise pathway. Surgery in children should always be optimized, and the most conservative surgical treatment possible should be considered.

POTENTIAL TREATMENTS MODALITIES

Potential treatment modalities include the following:
- Voice therapy with speech language pathologist: vocal hygiene and abuse reduction, hydration, increase/decrease glottal closure, decrease muscular tension, respiration, easy onset, improve coordination of respiration and phonation, resonance/voice placement, decrease ventricular phonation, raise/lower pitch, increase/decrease loudness, lower laryngeal placement, reinforce reflux treatment.
- Medical therapy and minimizing environmental factors: hydration, environmental allergies, allergic rhinitis (avoidance of antihistamines, use of intranasal steroid sprays), asthma (inhaled steroid preparations), GERD (basic GERD precautions, antacids, prokinetic drugs [cisapride], H_2-receptor antagonists, proton-pump inhibitors [omeprazole]).

- Surgical therapy when medical management/voice therapy fails: conservative excision of benign lesions, "cold" techniques, microlaryngeal instruments; avoidance of laser on true vocal folds; submucosal infusion technique, management of laryngeal papillomas, injection medialization laryngoplasty, nonselective recurrent laryngeal nerve reinnervation, destructive or expansion laryngeal framework surgery.

SUMMARY

Pediatric voice disorders remain a varied and challenging evolving field. Voice disorders in children are increasing being noted as a barrier to success in the school environment in terms of academic achievement and socialization. Significant advances over the past decade in evaluation, diagnosis, and management of pediatric voice disorders have improved both short-term and long-term outcomes for the dysphonic child.

Practitioners should have a thorough understanding of anatomy and physiology, how to accurately work up a pediatric voice disorder, and how to efficiently treat voice disorders. Comprehensive voice evaluation in children with subjective markers and objective markers is essential to properly assessing pediatric dysphonia. Diagnosis and treatment are best managed by a multidisciplinary team of otolaryngology, speech language pathology, and potentially pulmonology, gastroenterology, neurology, and others. Accurate diagnosis allows for effective treatment, which includes voice therapy, medical therapy, and/or surgical intervention as needed.

Further outcomes studies are needed to demonstrate the efficacy of the current and future comprehensive regimens (surgical, nonsurgical, combined) toward pediatric dysphonia in this new and evolving field.

CLINICS CARE POINTS

- Pediatric dysphonia is commonly underdiagnosed and may cause social isolation and impact a patient's academic, social, and emotional life.

- Subjective and objective measures can be used to best evaluate pediatric dysphonia in a combined visit to an otolaryngologist and a speech language pathologist. Typically, pediatric dysphonia is best managed with an experienced multidisciplinary team.

- Stroboscopy is a useful objective tool to identify causes of pediatric dysphonia and can evaluate motion as well as mucosal pathologic condition.

- Vocal fold motion impairment is the second most common congenital pathologic condition and can be unilateral or bilateral in nature.

- Benign vocal fold lesions are the most common cause of pediatric dysphonia, with vocal fold nodules the most common benign vocal fold lesion found.

- Functional voice disorders, although infrequent, may require in-depth understanding of the nature of the dysphonia, as there may be only subtle changes that dramatically affect the voice.

- Treatment of pediatric dysphonia can vary greatly and depends on the nature of the dysphonia. Treatment includes conservative treatment of observation, voice therapy, medical therapy and interventional treatment of injection medialization, surgical intervention, and laryngeal reinnervation.

- Deciding on when to operate on a dysphonic child greatly depends on the nature of the dysphonia, the maturity of the patient, and the ability of the child to undergo voice therapy preoperatively and postoperatively.

- General management of the pediatric airway is a balance of maintaining a good airway while maintaining a good voice. Optimizing airway and voice remains the quintessential challenge in the management of pediatric dysphonia.

DISCLOSURE

The authors have nothing to disclose.

REFERENCES

1. Carding PN, Roulstone S, Northstone K, et al. The prevalence of childhood dysphonia: a cross-sectional study. J Voice Dec 2006;20(4):623–30.
2. Connor NP, Cohen SB, Theis SM, et al. Attitudes of children with dysphonia. J Voice Mar 2008;22(2):197–209.
3. Prades JM, Dumollard JM, Duband S, et al. Lamina propria of the human vocal fold: histomorphometric study of collagen fibers. Surg Radiol Anat 2010;32(4): 377–82.
4. Markova D, Richer L, Pangelinan M, et al. Age- and sex-related variations in vocal-tract morphology and voice acoustics during adolescence. Horm Behav 2016;81:84–96.
5. Zur KB, Cotton S, Kelchner L, et al. Pediatric voice handicap index (pVHI): a new tool for evaluating pediatric dysphonia. Int J Pediatr Otorhinolaryngol 2007;71(1): 77–82.
6. Hartnick CJ. Validation of a pediatric voice quality of life instrument: the pediatric voice outcome survey. Arch Otolaryngol Head Neck Surg 2002;128:919–22.
7. Brandwein M, Abramson AL, Shikowitz MJ. Bilateral vocal cord paralysis following endotracheal intubation. Arch Otolaryngol Head Neck Surg 1986; 112(8):877–82.
8. Gorantla SC, Chan T, Shen I, et al. Current epidemiology of vocal cord dysfunction after congenital heart surgery in young infants. Pediatr Crit Care Med 2019; 20(9):817–25.
9. Zur KB, Carroll LM. Recurrent laryngeal nerve reinnervation in children: acoustic and endoscopic characteristics pre-intervention and post-intervention. A comparison of treatment options. Laryngoscope 2015;125(Suppl 11):S1–15. Epub 2015 Aug 8. Erratum in: Laryngoscope. 2017;127(2):E83.
10. Miyamoto RC, Cotton RT, Rope AF, et al. Association of anterior glottis webs with velocardiofacial syndrome (chromosome 22q11.2 deletion). Otolaryngol Head Neck Surg 2004;130(4):415–7.
11. Lawlor C, Balakrishnan K, Bottero S, et al. International Pediatric Otolaryngology Group (IPOG): juvenile-onset recurrent respiratory papillomatosis consensus recommendations. Int J Pediatr Otorhinolaryngol 2020;128:109697.
12. Matsuzaki H, Makiyama K, Hirai R, et al. Multi-year effect of human papillomavirus vaccination on recurrent respiratory papillomatosis. Laryngoscope 2020;130(2): 442–7.
13. Roy N. Functional dysphonia. Curr Opin Otolaryngol Head Neck Surg 2003;11: 144–8.
14. Campbell TF, Dollaghan CA, Yaruss JS. Disorders of language, phonology, fluency, and voice in children: indicators for referral. In: Bluestone CD, Stool SE, et al, editors. Pediatric otolaryngology. 4th Edition. Philadelphia, (PA): Saunders; 2003. p. 1773–87.

15. Goldenberg RL, Culhane JF, Iams JD, et al. Epidemiology and causes of preterm birth. Lancet 2008;371(9606):75–84.
16. Watters KF. Tracheostomy in infants and children. Respir Care 2017;62(6): 799–825.
17. de Alarcón A, Zacharias S, Oren L, et al. Endoscopic posterior cricoid reduction: a surgical method to improve posterior glottic diastasis. Laryngoscope 2019; 129(S2):S1–9.
18. Fritz MA, Rickert SM. Prevalence of voice disturbances in the pediatric craniofacial patient population. Otolaryngol Head Neck Surg 2016;154(6):1128–31.
19. Zoizner-Agar G, Rotsides JM, Shao Q, et al. Proton pump inhibitor administration in neonates and infants. Lack of consensus - an ASPO survey. Int J Pediatr Otorhinolaryngol 2020;137:110200.

Pediatric Dysphagia

Annie E. Moroco, MD[a], Nicole L. Aaronson, MD, MBA[a,b,*]

KEYWORDS

- Dysphagia • Pediatric • Swallow • Disorder • Feeding difficulties

KEY POINTS

- Dysphagia is a common finding in the pediatric population, particularly in at-risk infants, such as those born prematurely.
- Findings of refusal to feed, excessive time spent feeding, cough or emesis, and failure to thrive are all concerning for underlying dysphagia.
- A multidisciplinary team is useful in the work-up and management of feeding disorders, because it is important to assess medical and psychosocial concerns.
- Identified structural or medical causes of dysphagia alone should not eliminate the need for a thorough work-up if symptoms persist, because multifactorial disease is common.

INTRODUCTION

The process of enteral feeding involves intake of solid or liquid substance to support appropriate nutritional status, which is vital to maintain human health. More importantly in the pediatric population, adequate nutrition supports growth during integral phases of development. Difficulty with feeding is attributed to swallowing disorders of a variety of origins.[1] Appropriate identification and early intervention are necessary for successful outcomes in growth and development for children.

Normal Swallow Function

The typical swallow is a complex process that is divided into the oral phase, the pharyngeal phase, and the esophageal phase as a food bolus is transported through the mouth and into the stomach. The oral phase consists of preparatory and transit subphases, both under voluntary control in adults, but reflexive in infants. First, in the preparatory subphase, the food is moistened and manipulated to form a cohesive food bolus. This requires appropriate sensation and coordination of tongue, soft and hard palate, and adequate lip closure, which is not fully developed until approximately 6 months of age. The tongue then mobilizes the bolus into the oropharynx during the

[a] Department of Otolaryngology–Head & Neck Surgery, Thomas Jefferson University Sidney Kimmel School of Medicine, 111 South 11th Street, Philadelphia, PA 19107, USA; [b] Department of Surgery, Division of Pediatric Otolaryngology, Nemours Children's Hospital of Delaware, 1600 Rockland Road Wilmington, DE 19803, USA
* Corresponding author. Department of Surgery, Division of Pediatric Otolaryngology, Nemours Children's Hospital of Delaware, 1600 Rockland Road, Wilmington, DE 19803, USA
E-mail address: nicole.aaronson@nemours.org

Pediatr Clin N Am 69 (2022) 349–361
https://doi.org/10.1016/j.pcl.2021.12.005
0031-3955/22/© 2021 Elsevier Inc. All rights reserved.

transit subphase. The pharyngeal phase is under reflexive control to protect the airway from aspiration. Coordination and proper muscle functioning, including velopharyngeal mechanism, base of tongue, laryngeal and pharyngeal musculature for nasopharyngeal closure, laryngeal elevation, vocal fold adduction, and pharyngeal contracture to safely propel the food bolus into the esophagus, are vital for this phase. Movement to the esophageal phase of the swallow initiates peristalsis.[2]

Definition of Dysphagia

Dysphagia is defined simply as difficulty swallowing. This is in the form of a perceived or objective impairment causing an abnormal delay in the transition of the food bolus through the three phases of swallow. Because the pharynx is shared in breathing and swallowing, a disruption to one function can affect the other. Problems can arise in any single phase of swallow or globally. Long-term consequences of dysphagia can contribute to malnutrition and stunted developmental growth.

Swallow is detected in the fetus in the tenth week of gestation; however, the development of an organized suck-pause pattern is thought to develop in utero at 27 weeks and fully matures by 34 weeks.[3] Although the pattern develops early, the rhythm evolves from a 1:1 suck-swallow ratio initially to a 3:1 ratio, allowing for greater volume intake at birth.[2]

Neonates are obligate nasal breathers, in that the pharynx is functionally separated to allow for simultaneous airflow and swallow. Anatomically, the larynx lies superiorly allowing the epiglottis to interdigitate with the soft palate. This creates a respiratory pathway via the nares and a feeding pathway laterally via the piriform sinuses. This mechanism is required to coordinate the suck-swallow-breathe pattern required for feeding.

Epidemiology

Pediatric dysphagia is estimated to occur in less than 1% of the population.[4] Certain groups are at even higher risk of developing dysphagia, including children with neurologic deficits and history of prematurity.[5–7] The prevalence of dysphagia in premature infants is 10%, and when infants are simultaneously born with birth weight less than 1500 g, that estimate increases to nearly 25%.[8]

Common Presentation

Presenting symptoms of dysphagia vary based on age and pathologic cause. In the neonate, oral dysphagia may present as a poorly coordinated suck, whereas pharyngeal dysphagia may present with choking or reflux symptoms. Symptoms of concern may be noticed in the home. These include prolonged feeding time, posturing, or coughing with feeds, which may prompt a visit to the clinician who may further discover poor weight gain or recurrent lung infection. This presentation may vary in children of different age groups, and the assessment of children with feeding issues should include medical and psychosocial concerns.

DISCUSSION
Initial Work-up

When first assessing a patient for dysphagia, it is important to perform a thorough history and physical examination to include character of dysphagia, contributing factors, and associated symptoms. Important considerations include reflux behavior, regurgitation, recurrent respiratory illness, and personal or family history of atopy. Several scales to characterize dysphagia have been used in the adult population.[9] The Schedule for Oral-Motor Assessment and the Dysphagia Disorder Survey have been suggested as strong clinically validated scales to use in pediatric populations.[7,10,11]

A thorough physical examination of the head and neck is important when first evaluating these children. Findings of ankyloglossia or hypotonia may be readily apparent; however, other signs of cough or atopy should be investigated. Assessment should also include a neurologic examination.

A multidisciplinary coordinated effort is essential to the care of the child with dysphagia, and consultation with speech language pathology (SLP) is important in appropriate work-up and therapeutic management in many conditions. The SLP evaluation can include bedside swallow, where the problematic phase may be easily identified. Other common consultations may include pulmonology, gastroenterology, neurology, nutrition, and lactation specialists.

The modified barium swallow (MBS), also called the videofluoroscopic swallow study, can determine appropriate phase motility and assess safety of oral feeding. The MBS was first used in the 1950s and uses barium-dyed liquids of varying thickness to radiographically assess the swallow. Its utility is especially important in the assessment of silent aspiration; however, MBS is limited in its ability to assess the breastfeeding patient and the need for radiographic exposure. When concern arises for perforation or in the setting of recent surgery to the gastrointestinal tract, it is important to assess using a water-soluble agent. If there is high concern for aspiration, the MBS is performed using a contrast agent with low osmolarity, such as iopamidol, to protect the lungs from severe complication.

In contrast, the flexible endoscopic evaluation of swallowing is a more recent addition to the clinical toolbox and allows assessment of aspiration and laryngeal function under direct visualization without the need for radiation exposure. It is performed by an otolaryngologist in collaboration with SLP. The flexible nasopharyngolaryngoscope is introduced while the patient is fed different consistencies to assess anatomy and physiology of the swallow. The examination is often limited by tolerance of the scope. MBS and flexible endoscopic evaluation have advantages and limitations; they are often used in combination as complementary studies.[12]

Using these techniques as part of the initial work-up can typically narrow the potential causes of dysphagia. Based on the presumptive cause, further work-up can be done to achieve definitive diagnosis and determine treatment options. Other specific tests to consider include manometry, or further imaging, such as MRI, which is notably indicated when there is concern for neurologic cause. Procedural evaluation, which includes direct laryngoscopy, rigid bronchoscopy, and flexible scope examination, may be warranted. These surgical examinations can be coordinated to include flexible bronchoscopy with bronchoalveolar lavage and flexible esophagoscopy with biopsy, which may be done in coordination with a multidisciplinary team if desired.

Causes of Dysphagia

Nonstructural causes

It is important for the clinician to distinguish aversion from pathologic dysphagia. A child with oral aversion or a disorder in feeding behavior has the ability but is not willing to consume a food product. Subclinical oral aversions are thought to be prevalent in the population, with nearly one-half of children affected.[13] To diagnose behavioral aversion, it is important to involve the caregiver in the assessment for poor appetite or fear related to food selection or intake that cannot be explained by cultural practices or challenges with body image. Once other medical diagnoses are no longer considered, the patient should be referred for interdisciplinary feeding treatment.[14]

The exact cause of dysphagia may be difficult to ascertain, because it may often result from multifactorial comorbidities. We discuss a few of the nonstructural causes of dysphagia, which are commonly managed medically.

Premature infants are a unique population at higher risk for the development of dysphagia, because most infants begin to coordinate the suck-swallow-breathe pattern by 34 weeks gestation to begin appropriate feeding.[2,5] The origin of their feeding difficulty is often multifactorial, because delayed development of motor function including head control, tongue and palate mobility, and sensation contributing to laryngeal and gag reflexes can all play a role in dysphagia, and serve to further exacerbate any concomitant neural developmental delays. These infants are commonly those with complicated chronic lung and neurologic comorbidities.

Additionally, iatrogenic causes as in the case of prolonged intubation or tracheostomy can further contribute to difficulty feeding in these infants. Prolonged intubation can lead to incompetence at the level of the nasopharynx to the glottis, and when a tracheostomy tube is present, it can cause anatomic and functional changes to the swallow. Although most patients are able to resume an oral diet, some may not be able to do so, and the generation of a normal swallow is challenging and painful.[15]

Neuromuscular disorders encompass many diseases that can contribute to disruption in the coordination of appropriate swallow. The mechanism may be either direct pathology of muscle fibers or may involve nerve functioning. Hypotonia is the most prevalent symptom, and this low muscle tone can contribute to poor swallow and also cause aspiration and poor weight gain. Involvement of the central nervous system as in cerebral palsy, Arnold-Chiari malformations, and prior stroke contributes to the development of dysphagia in children.[7] Cerebral palsy is the most common neuromuscular condition seen in children, and there is significant overlap between this and prematurity, such that cerebral palsy is present in 20% of infants born before 26 weeks.[3] Several other neuromuscular conditions can contribute to dysphagia including microcephaly, hydrocephalus, congenital viral infection, seizure disorders, and traumatic brain injury. It is important to assess for neuromuscular conditions in addition to structural causes of dysphagia. For example, in infants with laryngomalacia and comorbid cerebral palsy, supraglottoplasty yields significantly poorer outcomes compared with those with only structural abnormality.[16]

Gastroesophageal reflux disease (GERD) is the symptomatic reflux of gastric contents. In the newborn, reflux is expected, and may even be considered normal when associated with emesis or regurgitation. Concerning symptoms of GERD include irritability, refusal to feed, stridor, hoarseness, posturing, or failure to thrive in an infant. In the older child, symptomatic GERD includes epigastric pain, globus sensation, odynophagia, and chest pain. Formal diagnosis made with esophageal pH testing or 24-hour multichannel intraluminal impedance may be performed. Although the classically described trial of antireflux medication may be diagnostic and therapeutic for the child, it is not currently recommended for neonates.[17,18]

The management of GERD is largely medical and classically performed by gastroenterology. Modification of feeds using thickeners is helpful in symptom management. If nutritional management is not sufficient, acid suppression medication may be used. In the neonate, proton pump inhibitors are used when reflux is causing erosive esophagitis. In extreme cases, surgical intervention in the form of fundoplication performed by general surgery may be necessary. Typically, surgical options are pursued if the child continues with severe complication while on medical management.[19]

Eosinophilic esophagitis is an inflammatory disease often associated with food allergies or other atopy. In addition to dysphagia, children often present with feeding intolerance, food impaction, choking during meals, emesis, and abdominal pain.

Tissue diagnosis demonstrating more than 15 eosinophils per high powered field is required; however, on esophagogastroduodenoscopy, the hallmark trachealization of the esophagus is often observed. Management often involves a multidisciplinary team that includes a gastroenterologist, an allergist, and a nutritionist. Treatment involves full changes in diet, such as an elemental diet or a food-elimination diet and medical treatment with proton pump inhibitors and topical glucocorticoids. Esophageal dilation may also be used in some cases.[20,21]

As a group, these conditions are commonly managed medically, and symptomatic improvement results after treatment of the underlying conditions, as in eosinophilic esophagitis and GERD. In multifactorial causes, the role of a multidisciplinary treatment team is important, particularly the role of the SLP in feeding therapy. The SLP can educate parents regarding appropriate pacing, positioning, and nipple selection for feeding. These feeding modifications can support improvement in the suck-swallow-breathe mechanism.

Structural causes

Nasal and nasopharyngeal. Several structural abnormalities in the upper aerodigestive tract can contribute to the development of dysphagia. Because newborns are obligate nasal breathers, congenital nasal obstruction can present as dysphagia with symptoms worsening during feedings and thus contributing to failure to thrive.

Choanal atresia is a congenital obstruction of the posterior nasal cavity, which can be occluded by membranous soft tissue, bone, or most commonly a combination bony-membranous. Bilateral only accounts for 30% of choanal atresia, and it should be suspected in the newborn with cyclical episodes of apnea with cyanosis resolved by crying. It may be suspected in the newborn where a catheter is unable to pass through the nasal passages. Formal evaluation with computed tomography is indicated. When diagnosed in the infant, evaluation for associated syndromes should be explored, most commonly CHARGE, but also Apert, Treacher Collins, and Crouzon. Early endoscopic surgical repair is vital in cases of bilateral choanal atresia. Unilateral choanal atresia is not usually associated with dysphagia and is repaired electively, and current recommendations encourage delay of at least 6 months or up to 2 years.[22]

When evaluating a nasal cause for dysphagia, it is important to distinguish choanal atresia from pyriform aperture stenosis. The pyriform aperture is the most anterior bony portion of the nasal airway and, when stenotic, can present in the infant. Formal diagnosis is made using computed tomography imaging, where the piriform aperture is found to be less than 11 mm in width. As seen in **Fig. 1**, this condition may be accompanied by central mega incisor, and when seen, evaluation of the brain for holoprosencephaly and pituitary abnormalities is indicated. Unlike bilateral choanal atresia, surgical intervention is not always imperative in the management of piriform aperture stenosis. Instead, medical therapy, such as topical decongestants, can often be prescribed until the infant is able to outgrow the restriction. Surgery should be considered when the child is unable to maintain appropriate weight gain. Surgical repair may require sublabial drill-out to enlarge the aperture. Supplemental nutrition may be required for a time following surgical correction as the neonate learns to coordinate the swallow.[22]

Adenoid hypertrophy can contribute to dysphagia in children. These children commonly present with hyponasal speech, chronic mouth breathing, and adenoid facies, which may also be seen in combination with tonsillar hypertrophy. Radiographic imaging is diagnostic, as shown in **Fig. 2**. Medical therapy can include topical steroid treatment; however, definitive management is surgical excision.[23]

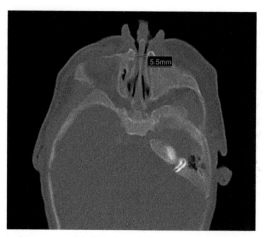

Fig. 1. Axial computed tomography showing piriform stenosis measured at 5.5 mm.

Oral and oropharyngeal. Ankyloglossia is a common consultation to the otolaryngologist and may contribute to dysphagia in the infant. Currently a topic of controversy in the surgical community, ankyloglossia limits mobility of the tongue. This is thought to contribute to poor latch and subsequent difficulty with suck-swallow-breathe leading to failure to thrive. Other symptoms commonly observed in ankyloglossia include aerophagia and leakage during feeding. Tethering may occur at various positions along the anteroposterior axis, and there is no current consensus on the role of surgery in these various groupings.[24] Frenotomy is the surgical intervention of choice. Although it is generally understood that neonates can tolerate this procedure at the bedside, older children may require a trip to the operating room. There is no clear consensus with respect to the exact age or other indications for operative intervention.[19] Evidence to support the role of frenotomy in improving dysphagia is minimal,

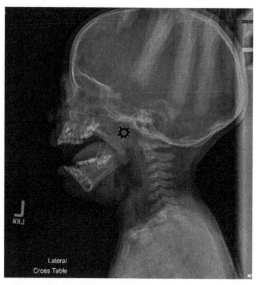

Fig. 2. Lateral neck radiograph showing adenoid hypertrophy. *Asterisk* denotes the adenoid pad.

and current literature suggests that surgical intervention may improve maternal pain with feeding without significant improvement in dysphagia.[25,26] Although ankyloglossia may be a contributor to dysphagia, it is important to assess for additional causes.

Craniofacial abnormalities may contribute to poor feeding, and most commonly cleft lip and palate refer to a spectrum of congenital malformations in craniofacial development. Often identified prenatally, these infants present with dysphagia and airway concerns immediately at birth because of the inability to create negative pressure. Inadequate feeding in these patients is a result of poor suction, excessive air intake, and velopharyngeal insufficiency leading to nasal regurgitation. The extent of cleft varies from unilateral to bilateral and incomplete to complete and correlates with symptom severity. Submucous cleft palate may often be a subclinical finding; however, it should be included in the differential for dysphagia because it can contribute to the development of nasal regurgitation and velopharyngeal insufficiency.[27] Depending on the specific type of cleft, patients may benefit from consultation with lactation specialists and SLP to optimize feeding technique. Cleft lip repair is typically performed around 3 months at his age. Nasoalveolar molding and such techniques as lip adhesion are sometimes used before definitive repair. Cleft palate repair may be performed in one to two stages. When done in two stages the soft palate is typically repaired between 3 and 8 months, whereas hard palate repair is delayed until 15 months or later.[28]

Compressive midline masses can contribute to the development of dysphagia at any age. These masses can acutely enlarge and in the pediatric neck, can quickly cause symptoms of dysphagia. Cystic masses along the alimentary tract include the vallecular cyst or ranula.[29] Further consideration is given to externally compressive masses, including the thyroglossal duct cyst, dermoid cyst, branchial cleft cyst, and thyroid mass. It is important to consider a malignancy when a distinct mass is found on clinical or radiographic examination.[30] Further consideration of lymphovascular malformation may be warranted in masses that episodically swell.[31]

Laryngeal. In the neonate, the epiglottis engages with the soft palate to support the suck-swallow-breathe sequence. When anatomic changes are present in the larynx, dysphagia is often a presenting symptom.

In laryngomalacia, the most common cause of stridor in infants, supraglottic structures collapse, which is acutely worsened during feeding, agitation, or when positioned supine. Nearly half of patients with laryngomalacia have feeding difficulty, and 10% of infants have severe complications, primarily failure to thrive.[32,33] The contribution to dysphagia is explained in many ways, including decreased laryngeal sensation, poor muscular tone, and difficulty coordinating the normal suck-swallow-breathe sequence because of increased work of breathing.[34]

Common symptoms seen in laryngomalacia include regurgitation, choking, and slow feedings, and these symptoms typically present within the first few weeks of life. The patient's symptoms commonly peak around 4 to 6 months of age, and symptoms may last until age 1 or 2 years. Diagnosis requires visualization using flexible nasopharyngolaryngoscopy, and the diagnosis encompasses the collapse of many supraglottic structures, including shortened aryepiglottic folds, hooded arytenoid cartilages, and the classic omega-shaped epiglottis. Although there is an obvious structural component, the cause may be multifactorial and further complicated by neurologic influence. Furthermore, the cyclical relationship with GERD causing inflammation and decreased sensation is thought to exacerbate laryngomalacia.[33,35]

Although commonly self-limited, when dysphagia is severe enough to cause failure to thrive, consideration of surgical intervention is warranted. Supraglottoplasty is a procedure that divides aryepiglottic folds and additionally can remove redundant arytenoid tissue, as shown in **Fig. 3**. Proper assessment postoperatively is important because aspiration can develop as a consequence of surgical intervention. Supraglottic stenosis and altered sensation to the region may increase risk of aspiration, particularly observed in children with aspiration preoperatively.[36] Evaluation of the holistic patient is important when assessing the role that surgery may play in laryngomalacia, because evidence suggests supraglottoplasty failure is more likely in children with significant medical comorbidity.[34,37]

Vocal fold paralysis or paresis may be secondary to birth trauma, Chiari malformation, other neurologic abnormalities, prior surgery, or idiopathic. Although paralysis describes true immobility, vocal cord paresis is used to describe any weakened cord motion. Although not all children with vocal fold immobility experience aspiration, it can contribute to symptomatic dysphagia in up to 50% of patients.[38] Unilateral symptomatic vocal fold immobility commonly presents with weak cry or hoarseness in the older child, in addition to dysphagia, whereas bilateral vocal fold immobility is classically present in the newborn with audible stridor. Diagnosis uses the nasopharyngolaryngoscope to examine vocal fold mobility. If no obvious cause for the immobility is identified, imaging along the course of the recurrent laryngeal nerve from the skull base to the aortic arch should be pursued.

Depending on cause, spontaneous resolution may occur in 25% of patients within 6 months. Furthermore, independent of return in vocal fold function, resolution of dysphagia may occur spontaneously.[38] With age and therapy, patients with unchanged vocal fold immobility may learn to adjust their behavior to safely swallow without experiencing dysphagia, even in children with bilateral vocal fold paralysis.[39]

Surgical intervention may be warranted in the patient with persistent vocal fold paralysis, and in the child with dysphagia, injection laryngoplasty is commonly the initial treatment. This uses an absorbable material, such as carboxymethyl cellulose, which has effect for anywhere from 1 to 6 months. If dysphagia persists, formal medialization thyroplasty or reinnervation procedures may be indicated in certain cases, taking into consideration patient age, prognosis, and cause. In children with bilateral vocal fold paralysis, intervention depends on positioning of the cords. If cords remain in an abducted position, it is possible that no respiratory intervention is needed but aspiration may be more likely. When the cords remain in an adducted position, which is more common, respiratory compromise is more likely. This may result in posterior cordotomy, vocal cord lateralization, or tracheostomy to maintain the airway.[40]

Laryngeal cleft is the failure in development of tracheoesophageal septum and may be present in the child with dysphagia with stridor and frequent aspiration events

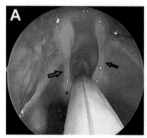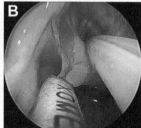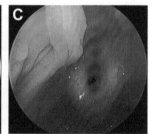

Fig. 3. (*A*) Tight aryepiglottic folds in the setting of laryngomalacia. *Arrows* point to left and right aryepiglottic folds. *Asterisk* denotes left arytenoid. Right arytenoid obscured by endotracheal tube. (*B*) Release of the left aryepiglottic fold after cutting with laryngeal scissors. (*C*) Postoperative view after cutting of bilateral aryepiglottic folds and trimming of the redundant arytenoid mucosa.

leading to recurrent pneumonia. It is uncommon for these children to be diagnosed as infants; instead, the diagnosis is classically made in the older child with recurrent pulmonary infections and feeding difficulties. Occasionally, the patient requires a nasogastric or gastronomy tube, but this is uncommon. The laryngeal cleft requires operative diagnosis, during which the interarytenoid groove is palpated to determine the degree of cleft. Using the Benjamin classification system, type 1 involves the supraglottic interarytenoid cleft above the level of the vocal fold, type 2 extends into the cricoid cartilage, type 3 into the cervical trachea, and type 4 into the thoracic trachea.[41]

Diagnosis can often be delayed in patients with type 1 and type 2 clefts, even when symptomatic, because a high level of clinical suspicion is required.[42] Patients may be managed medically using thickeners and feeding strategies to allow for growth with great success. Half of patients undergoing conservative management report symptom improvement.[43] However, if dysphagia persists, management in the form of injection laryngoplasty or endoscopic repair is indicated. Injection of a filler may be diagnostic and therapeutic before definitive surgical repair. Endoscopic surgical repair is preferred for types 1 and 2 (**Fig. 4**). Open surgical intervention is preferred for types 3 and 4.[44]

Tracheal and esophageal. In tracheoesophageal fistula, there is a developmental failure in the formation of distinct trachea and esophagus that can include various combinations of atresia or fistula. Many present as neonates with episodic cyanosis; children with other variations may present later in life with recurrent aspiration pneumonia. Diagnosis classically involves a combination of imaging and direct visualization with bronchoscopy and esophagoscopy. These are typically managed surgically via thoracotomy, transcervical approach, endoscopic approach, or minimally invasive thoracoscopic approach.[45]

Achalasia is caused by tonic contraction of the upper esophageal sphincter with only intermittent relaxation, which can contribute to dysphagia. Children present with episodes of coughing, choking, and gagging during meals, often worsened with liquid more than solids. In the case of upper esophageal sphincter cause, diagnosis is made using MBS to reveal a cricopharyngeal bar, although manometry can also be used to confirm tonic activation of the cricopharyngeal muscle. When the lower esophageal sphincter is involved, the MBS classically demonstrates a dilated esophagus with a "bird beak" appearance distally. Achalasia is managed via Botox injections to the upper esophageal sphincter or cricopharyngeal myotomy.[46]

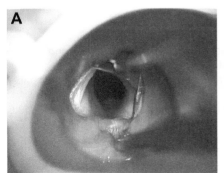 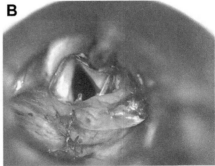

Fig. 4. (*A*) Endoscopic suturing of a type 2 laryngeal cleft. (*B*) Postoperative view after suturing of the laryngeal cleft.

Extrinsic vascular compression may contribute to dysphagia and tracheomalacia. Dysphagia lusoria is a term used to describe vascular compression of the esophagus by an aberrant right subclavian artery. Such vascular compression commonly presents as biphasic stridor and diagnosis is apparent on imaging demonstrating retroesophageal right subclavian artery. When operative aerodigestive evaluation is pursued, bronchoscopy reveals a pulsatile posterior tracheal wall compression. Definitive treatment requires surgical intervention with a pediatric cardiothoracic surgeon.[47]

Multifactorial causes

Follow-up after surgical intervention is important for these children even when a structural cause for dysphagia is identified and treated, because there may be further underlying multifactorial etiologies aside from the obvious. When a surgical intervention alone is not the solution, the importance of involving a multidisciplinary team must be stressed. The role of therapists and medical collaborators in identifying and managing complex neurologic causes of dysphagia, in addition to muscular and anatomic causes, should be highly valued. It is also important to consider systemic causes including rheumatologic conditions and adverse effects of medication.

SUMMARY

Overall, feeding difficulty is a common problem in the pediatric population. It is important to differentiate a true pathologic cause of dysphagia from an oral aversion. Diagnosis and management of dysphagia should involve a multidisciplinary team, because etiologies can include structural and nonstructural causes.

CLINICS CARE POINTS

- Findings on history and physical examination concerning for clinical dysphagia include limited interest in feeding, excessive time spent feeding, emesis or coughing during feeds, and failure to thrive.

- Diagnosis should be made in collaboration with a multidisciplinary team, including speech language pathology, gastroenterology, pulmonology, dietetics, and behavioral psychology.

- Identified structural or medical causes of dysphagia alone should not eliminate the need for a thorough work-up if symptoms persist, because multifactorial disease is common.

DISCLOSURE

The authors have nothing to disclose.

REFERENCES

1. Dodrill P, Gosa MM. Pediatric dysphagia: physiology, assessment, and management. Ann Nutr Metab 2015;66(Suppl 5):24–31.
2. Raol N, Schrepfer T, Hartnick C. Aspiration and dysphagia in the neonatal patient. Clin Perinatol 2018;45:645–60.
3. Kakodkar K, Schroeder JW. Pediatric dysphagia. Pediatr Clin North Am 2013;60: 969–77.
4. Bhattacharyya N. The prevalence of pediatric voice and swallowing problems in the United States. Laryngoscope 2015;125:746–50.
5. Lefton-Greif MA, Arvedson JC. Pediatric feeding and swallowing disorders: state of health, population trends, and application of the international classification of functioning, disability, and health. Semin Speech Lang 2007;28:161–5.

6. Hawdon J, Beauregard N, Slattery J, et al. Identification of neonates at risk of developing feeding problems in infancy. Dev Med Child Neurol 2000;42:235–9.

7. Benfer KA, Weir KA, Boyd RN. Clinimetrics of measures of oropharyngeal dysphagia for preschool children with cerebral palsy and neurodevelopmental disabilities: a systematic review. Dev Med Child Neurol 2012;54:784–95.

8. Jadcherla S. Dysphagia in the high-risk infant: potential factors and mechanisms. Am J Clin Nutr 2016;103:622S–8S.

9. Sallum RAA, Duarte AF, Cecconello I. Analytic review of dysphagia scales. Arq Bras Cir Dig 2012;25:279–82.

10. Ko MJ, Kang MJ, Ko KJ, et al. Clinical usefulness of schedule for oral-motor assessment (SOMA) in children with dysphagia. Ann Rehabil Med 2011;35:477–84.

11. Sheppard JJ, Hochman R, Baer C. The dysphagia disorder survey: validation of an assessment for swallowing and feeding function in developmental disability. Res Dev Disabil 2014;35:929–42.

12. Brady S, Donzelli J. The modified barium swallow and the functional endoscopic evaluation of swallowing. Otolaryngol Clin North Am 2013;46:1009–22.

13. Edwards S, Davis AM, Ernst L, et al. Interdisciplinary strategies for treating oral aversions in children. J Parenter Enteral Nutr 2015;39:899–909.

14. Estrem HH, Pados BF, Park J, et al. Feeding problems in infancy and early childhood: evolutionary concept analysis. J Adv Nurs 2017;73:56–70.

15. Luu K, Belsky MA, Dharmajan H, et al. Dysphagia in pediatric patients with tracheostomy. Ann Otol Rhinol Laryngol 2021. https://doi.org/10.1177/00034894211025179. 34894211025179.

16. Durvasula VSPB, Lawson BR, Bower CM, et al. Supraglottoplasty outcomes in neurologically affected and syndromic children. JAMA Otolaryngol Head Neck Surg 2014;140:704–11.

17. Barfield E, Parker MW. Management of pediatric gastroesophageal reflux disease. JAMA Pediatr 2019;173:485–6.

18. Rosen R, Vandenplas Y, Singendonk M, et al. Pediatric gastroesophageal reflux clinical practice guidelines: joint recommendations of the North American Society for Pediatric Gastroenterology, Hepatology, and Nutrition and the European Society for Pediatric Gastroenterology, Hepatology, and Nutrition. J Pediatr Gastroenterol Nutr 2018;66:516–54.

19. Duncan DR, Larson K, Rosen RL. Clinical aspects of thickeners for pediatric gastroesophageal reflux and oropharyngeal dysphagia. Curr Gastroenterol Rep 2019;21(7):30.

20. Furuta GT, Katzka DA. Eosinophilic esophagitis. N Engl J Med 2015;373(17):1640–8.

21. Moreddu E, Rizzi M, Adil E, et al. International Pediatric Otolaryngology Group (IPOG) consensus recommendations: diagnosis, pre-operative, operative and post-operative pediatric choanal atresia care. Int J Pediatr Otorhinolaryngol 2019;123:151–5.

22. Serran TL, Pfeilsticker L, Silva V, et al. Newborn nasal obstruction due to congenital nasal pyriform aperture stenosis. Allergy Rhinol 2016;17(1):37–41.

23. Lawlor CM, Choi S. Diagnosis and management of pediatric dysphagia: a review. JAMA Otolaryngol Head Neck Surg 2020;146(2):183–91.

24. Messner AH, Walsh J, Rosenfeld RM, et al. Clinical consensus statement: ankyloglossia in children. Otolaryngol Head Neck Surg 2020;162:597–611.

25. Muldoon K, Gallagher L, McGuinness D, et al. Effect of frenotomy on breastfeeding variables in infants with ankyloglossia (tongue-tie): a prospective before and after cohort study. BMC Pregnancy Childbirth 2017;17:373.
26. Francis DO, Krishnaswami S, McPheeters M. Treatment of ankyloglossia and breastfeeding outcomes: a systematic review. Pediatrics 2015;135:e1458–66.
27. Moss AL, Jones K, Pigott RW. Submucous cleft palate in the differential diagnosis of feeding difficulties. Arch Dis Child 1990;65:182–4.
28. Arosarena OA. Cleft lip and palate. Otolaryngol Clin North Am 2007;40(1):27–60.
29. Olojede ACO, Ogudana OM, Emeka CI, et al. Plinging ranula: surgical management of case series and the literature review. Clin Case Rep 2017;6(1):109–14.
30. Mattioni J, Azari S, Hoover T, et al. A cross-sectional evaluation of outcomes of pediatric thyroglossal duct cyst excision. ORL J Otorhinolaryngol Relat Spec 2021;29:1–8.
31. Johnston DR, Donaldson J, Cahill AM. New onset dysphagia and pulmonary aspiration following sclerotherapy for a complex cervical venolymphatic malformation in an infant case report and review of the literature. Int J Pediatr Otorhinolaryngol 2019;128:109694.
32. Ayari S, Aubertin G, Girschig H, et al. Pathophysiology and diagnostic approach to laryngomalacia in infants. Eur Ann Otorhinolaryngol Head Neck Dis 2012;129: 257–63.
33. Simons JP, Greenberg LL, Mehta DK, et al. Laryngomalacia and swallowing function in children. Laryngoscope 2016;126:478–84.
34. Carter J, Rahbar R, Brigger M, et al. International Pediatric ORL Group (IPOG) laryngomalacia consensus recommendations. Int J Pediatr Otorhinolaryngol 2016;86:256–61.
35. Thompson DM. Abnormal sensorimotor integrative function of the larynx in congenital laryngomalacia: a new theory of etiology. Laryngoscope 2007;117(6 Pt 2 Suppl 114):1–33.
36. Richter GT, Wootten CT, Rutter MJ, et al. Impact of supraglottoplasty on aspiration in severe laryngomalacia. Ann Otol Rhinol Laryngol 2009;118:259–66.
37. Preciado D, Zalzal G. A systematic review of supraglottoplasty outcomes. Arch Otolaryngol Head Neck Surg 2012;138:718–21.
38. Jabbour J, Martin T, Beste D, et al. Pediatric vocal fold immobility: natural history and the need for long-term follow-up. JAMA Otolaryngol Head Neck Surg 2014; 140:428–33.
39. Hsu J, Tibbetts KM, Wu D, et al. Swallowing function in pediatric patients with bilateral vocal fold immobility. Int J Pediatr Otorhinolaryngol 2017;93:37–41.
40. Butskiy O, Mistry B, Chadha N. Surgical interventions for pediatric unilateral vocal cord paralysis: a systematic review. JAMA Otolaryngol Head Neck Surg 2015; 141:654–60.
41. Benjamin B, Inglis A. Minor congenital laryngeal clefts: diagnosis and classification. Ann Otol Rhinol Laryngol 1989;98:417–20.
42. Reddy P, Byun YJ, Downs J, et al. Presentation and management of type 1 laryngeal clefts: a systematic review and meta-analysis. Int J Pediatr Otorhinolaryngol 2020;138:110370.
43. Timashpolsky A, Schild SD, Ballard DP, et al. Management of type 1 laryngeal clefts: a systematic review and meta-analysis. Otolaryngol Head Neck Surg 2021;164:489–500.
44. Yeung JC, Balakrishnan K, Cheng ATL, et al. International Pediatric Otolaryngology Group: consensus guidelines on the diagnosis and management of type I laryngeal clefts. Int J Pediatr Otorhinolaryngol 2017;101:51–6.

45. Kennedy AA, Hart CK, de Alarcon A, et al. Slide tracheoplasty for repair of complex tracheosopghageal fistulas. Laryngoscope 2021;10:1002.

46. Marchica C, Zawawi F, Daniel SJ. Management of cricopharyngeal achalasia in an 8-month child using endoscopic cricopharyngeal myotomy. Int J Pediatr Otorhinolaryngol 2017;101:137–40.

47. Nelson JS, Hurtado CG, Wearden PD. Surgery for dysphagia lusoria in children. Ann Thorac Surg 2020;109(2):131–3.

Pediatric Salivary Gland Disease

James Brett Chafin, MD[a],*, Leith Bayazid, MD[b]

KEYWORDS

- Pediatric • Salivary gland • Sialorrhea • Sialadenitis • Sialendoscopy

KEY POINTS

- Salivary stones are rare in children but may cause chronic sialadenitis.
- Sialendoscopy has emerged as the leading diagnostic and often therapeutic intervention for recurrent and chronic pediatric sialadenitis.
- Mumps has historically been the most common form of sialadenitis diagnosed in children internationally.
- Juvenile recurrent parotitis is the second most common form of sialadenitis in the pediatric population.
- Salivary gland tumors are very uncommon in children, representing less than 5% of salivary malignancies.

INTRODUCTION

The salivary glands develop as outgrowths of the oral epithelium, which expand as solid nests of cells into the underlying mesenchyme. [1–4] The parotid analog develops at 4 weeks of gestation, followed by the submandibular and sublingual primordia between 6 and 8 weeks. These cores undergo extensive branching, enlarge, and canalize to develop lumina. The enveloping mesenchyme divides the developing glands into lobules and forms a capsule.[5] The parotid glands are unique among the other salivary glands because they contain intraglandular lymph nodes and lymphatic tissue (**Fig. 1**). The parotid gland is the last of the glands to encapsulate, occurring after the development of the lymphatic system, resulting in entrapment of the lymphatics within the gland.[6]

Saliva is of paramount importance to every function for which the oral cavity is responsible. Saliva contains enzymes such as amylase and lipase, which aid in the

[a] Department of Pediatric Otolaryngology—Head & Neck Surgery, Nemours Children's Health System, 807 Childrens Way 4th Floor, Jacksonville, FL 32207, USA; [b] Department of Otolaryngology—Head and Neck Surgery, University of South Florida College of Medicine, 12901 Bruce B. Downs Boulevard, MDC 73, Tampa, FL 33612, USA
* Corresponding author.
E-mail address: Brett.Chafin@Nemours.org

Pediatr Clin N Am 69 (2022) 363–380
https://doi.org/10.1016/j.pcl.2022.01.004
0031-3955/22/© 2022 Elsevier Inc. All rights reserved.

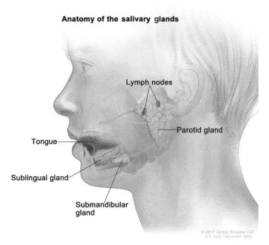

Anatomy of the salivary glands

Lymph nodes

Parotid gland

Tongue

Sublingual gland

Submandibular gland

© 2017 Terese Winslow LLC
U.S. Govt. has certain rights

Fig. 1. Anatomic locations of the 3 paired major salivary glands. There are lymphatic channels and nodes within the parotid gland. *Borrowed* with permission from Terese Winslow LLC.

digestion of food; in addition, it assists in the sensation of taste and in lubrication of the oral cavity.[7] Saliva aids in the proper articulation and modulation of speech; it also has antimicrobial properties, containing secretory IgA, mucins, and lactoferrin. Saliva balances the oral flora, aiding in maintaining the steady neutral pH of the oral cavity.[8] By continuously irrigating the oral cavity surfaces, saliva is important in the control of biofilms, preventing increased bacterial growth, recurrent infections, and erosion of the gingiva and teeth.[9]

The daily secretion of saliva ranges between 750 and 900 mL in children and increases to approximately 1 to 1.5 L of saliva in adults.[10] Excretion into the oral cavity is mainly ensured by the 3 paired major salivary glands. The parotid gland is the largest; its secretion is transmitted through the parotid duct, which enters the oral cavity at the level of the second maxillary molar. The submandibular gland and duct are located on the inner surface of the mandible, whereas the sublingual gland is embedded in the mucous membrane of the floor of the mouth and has a main duct with several minor ducts. The major glands are responsible for 90% of salivary secretion.[11] Apart from mealtimes, approximately 75% of saliva is produced by the submandibular glands as a mixture of serous and mucinous fluid, whereas 20% is produced by the parotid glands, which produce a serous, protein-rich (amylase) secretion. Saliva's major function is to break down complex carbohydrates.[11] With chewing, the ratio becomes reversed.[10] The regulation of this production is controlled by the autonomic nervous system: its quantity controlled by the parasympathetic system and its quality by the sympathetic system.

CONGENITAL SALIVARY ISSUES
Aplasia and Hypoplasia

Absence of the major salivary glands is very rare and may affect one or more gland. The cause is unknown but possibly related to a defect in early intrauterine development. This condition may be isolated or associated with other abnormalities including branchial and lacrimal anomalies.[12] Remaining glands may appear hypertrophied.

First Brachial Cleft Cyst

These cysts form as a result of incomplete fusion of the cleft between the first and second branchial arches; they are often asymptomatic until they present with infection with recurrent gland swelling or drainage into the external auditory canal.[13] Type I cysts may appear as an area of swelling near the ear, whereas type II must be considered with recurrent parotid abscesses.

OBSTRUCTIVE DISORDERS

With hundreds of minor salivary glands present in the oral cavity, patients may experience blockage with a resultant mucocele. These benign mucous-retention cysts of the oral cavity are often minimally symptomatic. When found on the floor of mouth or involving the sublingual gland, they are called ranulas. If a ranula persistently grows and falls below the floor of mouth, it is called a plunging ranula. The mucocele and ranula, collectively referred to as a mucous escape reaction, are most frequently diagnosed in the first or second decade of life. For the ranula, some investigators have recommended a 6-month observation period, after which time, patients should undergo excision if not resolved.[14] However, Seo and colleagues[15] found observation only allowed for an increase in size, and because none resolved, they recommended surgery with simultaneous excision of associated sublingual gland as first-line therapy given low morbidity.

SIALORRHEA

The constant secretion and swallowing of saliva requires a coordinated series of orofacial sensory and motor systems. This regulated act of swallowing is modulated by respiration. Sialorrhea (more commonly referred to as drooling) is defined as spillage of saliva due to either excessive production (primary sialorrhea) or decreased frequency of swallowing (secondary sialorrhea). Patients may present with anterior drooling, posterior drooling, or both. Anterior drooling is defined as saliva spilled from the mouth that is clearly visible, whereas posterior drooling occurs when saliva spills into the oropharynx with associated consequences of chronic aspiration and lung disease. Between 15 and 18 months of age, as the orofacial skeleton and swallowing mechanism matures, sialorrhea tends to resolve in children without neuromuscular comorbidities. Neuromuscular disorders may have an impact on this maturation process causing drooling to persist, and continuation beyond the fourth year is regarded as pathologic.[16] Consequences include sores on patients' lips and chins, a constant need for bibs for skin and clothing protection, required frequent changing of clothes, and difficulty sharing saturated toys, all resulting in child alienation, and in more severe cases, dehydration and aspiration pneumonia.[17]

Cerebral palsy (CP) describes a group of permanent disorders of the development of movement and posture, causing activity limitations. The condition is associated with poor oromotor control, and abnormalities in the deglutition reflex, as well as reduced intraoral sensitivities.[10] CP is the most common cause of persistent drooling in the pediatric population with a prevalence that ranges from 37% to 58%.[18,19]

Clinical examination should focus attention on proper function of facial, lingual, and soft palate motor activity and especially to muscle tone, head posturing, and any obstructive anatomic concerns, including dental malposition and occlusal disturbances. This condition is best addressed with a multidisciplinary team with the goal of clarifying the underlying condition and directing proper treatment.[16] Options for treatment include behavioral, pharmacologic, and surgical interventions. Behavioral approaches are based on physiotherapy and speech therapy and require proper motivation and a large time investment.[20] Pharmacotherapy with anticholinergics may cause dry mouth, blurred vision, confusion, somnolence, restlessness, and urinary retention. Thus, newer focus has been placed on botulinum toxin (BoNT) injection and surgical options. Little and colleagues[21] suggested an evidence-based stepwise approach to the drooling child involving the following stages:

1. Review posture and positioning
2. Oral awareness and oral motor skills training
3. Orthodontic evaluation/treatment
4. Pharmacotherapy
5. Botulinum injection
6. Surgical intervention

The early stages involve focus on positioning such as working with proper wheelchairs, addressing nasal obstruction that may be requiring mouth breathing, and dental evaluations to address caries or malocclusion. Speech therapy should be trialed for at least 6 months before surgical consideration. Patients with sialorrhea should undergo a screening for their swallowing ability by an appropriate therapist and may include radiographic and/or endoscopic examination. Functional dysphagia therapy may reduce the risk of aspiration and can use feedback techniques and kinesio-taping to improve spontaneous swallowing and saliva management.[16] These methods may be severely limited due to lack of cooperative skills in this patient population. Orthodontic approaches may aid in resolving malocclusive conditions.

Medical Management of Sialorrhea

Medical treatment aims to inhibit salivary secretion through anticholinergic/antagonist drugs; these include atropine, scopolamine, and glycopyrrolate, which have the advantage of inducing weaker central nervous system side effects.[16]

In 2001, Jongerius and colleagues[22] published the first case study on children with CP with sialorrhea treated with BoNT. BoNT is a potent neurotoxin produced by the *Clostridium botulinum* bacterium that blocks the presynaptic release of acetylcholine in the parasympathetic ganglia.[16] The blockade is only temporary because new nerves grow to create new neural connections.[23] The effects last 3 to 4 months, with a peak effect at 2 to 8 weeks postinjection.[16] Intraglandular injection of BoNT into the larger salivary glands blocks neurogenic control of salivary secretion. To reduce saliva secretion under conditions of both resting and stimulation, a review by Jost and colleagues[16] determined synchronous injection into the submandibular and parotid glands to be essential. Dosage for children has not achieved consensus. Studies including a meta-analysis from 2014 recommended using ultrasound guidance and injecting botulinum toxin A at 2 U/kg (1 mL/100 U) divided equally among all 4 glands.[10]

Alvarengo and colleagues[24] reported the efficacy of BoNT injections and found it to be minimally invasive treatment with few complications. Most favorable results were noted at 3 months after injection with requirement for reinjection becoming apparent at around 6 months. A systematic review of BoNT in the CP population by Rodwell and colleagues[25] found it to be an effective temporary treatment of sialorrhea with reduction of bibs per day, reduced score on Drooling Impact Scale, and Drooling Frequency and Severity.

The performance of injections under ultrasound guidance is recommended to help decrease the risk of dysphagia from toxin diffusion to the surrounding musculature and tissue with the majority in the pediatric population being performed under general anesthesia.[16,18] Side effects have reported to range from 2% to 41% and included dry mouth in 8% to 9%, dysphagia in 4%, and rarely pneumonia.[16,25] The mechanism for swallow and speech difficulties after injection may be related to the local diffusion of BoNT into the surrounding musculature, change in saliva properties, or systemic effect of BoNT.

Surgical Management of Sialorrhea

Surgical interventions for drooling may be considered when conservative measures, medical therapies, and/or BoNT injections fail to improve to be effective. Options vary from duct relocation or ligation to gland removal with varying degrees of success.

Salivary Duct Ligation

The concurrent ligation of the parotid and submandibular ducts has been described as first-line surgical management. The surgical simplicity, lack of external skin incision, and avoidance of nerve injury make it an attractive option. Success rates vary from 30% to 100% with recurrence rates ranging from 0% to 69% anywhere from 3.5 to 9 months postoperatively.[23] Studies are challenging to compare because the procedure may range from 2 to all 4 of the ducts ligated and may include additional procedures. El-Hakim and colleagues[26] noted benefits in reducing aspiration especially when all 4 ducts were ligated. Complications include xerostomia, gland infection and swelling, aspiration pneumonia, delayed resumption of oral feeding, and ranula formation.[23,27]

Salivary Duct Relocation

As the submandibular gland produces 70% of the resting salivary output, it is an obvious target for surgical intervention for saliva diversion. Submandibular duct relocation has been shown to be effective in up to 80% of children who have safe swallow.[23] The prospective study by Kok and colleagues[27] demonstrated a consistent and persistent reduction in drooling with reduced daily care. The surgery involves bilateral relocation of the submandibular ducts to the inferior pole of the palatine tonsil. Any concern for aspiration necessitates a formal preoperative swallow evaluation. A study by Sousa and colleagues[17] demonstrated a reduction in number of bibs a day with most caregivers being satisfied with results.

Salivary Gland Excision

With the effectiveness of 4-duct ligation unclear and contraindication of duct relocation in the setting of aspiration, bilateral submandibular gland excision is another potential intervention for the management of sialorrhea. Delsing and colleagues[28] reported 63% subjective success rate (>50% reduction in baseline) with gland excision. Risks include postoperative bleeding, xerostomia, and injury to marginal mandibular, lingual, and hypoglossal nerves. Gland excision with parotid duct ligation reduces both resting salivary flow and mastication-induced salivation and has been associated with an 83% reduction of drooling according to caregivers.[29] Intraoral submandibular gland excision has been reported by reducing risk of scarring and nerve injury. Reed and colleagues[30] performed a meta-analysis of the surgical management of drooling in 2009, and the overall success rate for all procedures was 81.6%. Bilateral SMGE with parotid duct rerouting was highest in subjective success at 87.8% and 4-duct ligation alone was lowest at 64.1%. However, these studies were generally of low quality and suffer from significant heterogeneity.[30]

Future Needs

Data on management of sialorrhea remains relatively limited for all interventions. BoNT is supported as a therapeutic option, and those who fail may warrant surgical intervention. Further research for pediatric protocols for BoNT injection focusing on dosage, effectiveness, and comparison with other forms of treatment are needed.

For surgical interventions, the current state of evidence is also low with only a small number of high-quality trials. Future studies are needed to address safety, compare efficacy, and develop a clear format for reporting adverse events as well as outcomes measures.

PEDIATRIC SIALADENITIS

Sialadenitis is defined as inflammation of a salivary gland. Pediatric sialadenitis accounts for 10% of all salivary gland disease with viral parotitis and juvenile recurrent parotitis (JRP) being the 2 most common causes.[31] Inflammatory disorders of the salivary glands may be infectious or noninfectious. See **Box 1** for a list of causes.

Infectious

Infectious disorders may involve the parenchyma of the salivary glands as a sialadenitis or the intrasalivary gland lymph nodes, as occurs in *Mycobacterium tuberculosis*

Box 1
Causes of infections and inflammatory sialadenitis

Viral
  Paramyxovirus (mumps)
  Epstein-Barr virus
  Parainfluenza
  HIV
  Coxsackie A and B
  Influenza A
  Cytomegalovirus

Bacterial
  Staphylococcus aureus
  Streptococcus viridians
  Haemophilus influenzae
  Peptostreptococcus spp
  Streptococcus pneumoniae
  Escherichia coli
  Bacteroides
  Actinomyces
  Bartonella henselae (cat-scratch disease)
  Mycobacterium tuberculosis
  Nontuberculous mycobacteria

Noninfectious/immune
  Sjögren syndrome
  Juvenile rheumatoid arthritis
  IgA deficiency
  Sarcoidosis

Traumatic
  Penetrating or blunt trauma
  Radiation
  Obstruction due to mass or stone

or nontuberculous mycobacterium. Infectious disorders more commonly affect a single gland in bacterial conditions and multiple glands in viral. Noninfectious inflammatory disease tends to involve multiple salivary glands as in Sjögren syndrome and sarcoidosis.[32]

Acute sialadenitis is most often caused by the paramyxovirus (mumps), although incidence has declined worldwide as a result of vaccination with an effectiveness approaching 90%.[31] Acute sialadenitis is a systemic illness that affects the salivary glands without producing purulence. Patients may also experience pain, fever, headache, and malaise. Serologic assays are useful in confirming diagnosis. Bacterial sialadenitis most commonly occurs in the parotid glands. Acute suppurative parotitis can develop from aerobic or anaerobic pathogens; they are likely the results of diminished salivary flow with ascending infection from the oral cavity or transient bacteremia.[31] The most common presenting symptoms of acute sialadenitis are swelling, pain, fever, trismus, and erythema overlying the affected gland. Symptoms are often unilateral; in bilateral cases, symptoms are often worse on one side. The opening of the duct may be erythematous and edematous, possibly with purulent fluid expressed with palpation. In the submandibular gland, infection may result in swelling in the floor of mouth and possibly respiratory distress. Purulent drainage through the duct is generally present, and the most common pathogens are Staphylococcus aureus and streptococcal species.[31] Other pathogens are listed in **Box 1**. Concern for abscess formation should be evaluated with imaging.

Chronic sialadenitis may also be due to immune deficiency (IgA), autoimmune disease such as Sjögren syndrome, and chronic viral conditions (human immunodeficiency virus [HIV]). Parotid gland enlargement is estimated to occur in up to 10% of HIV-infected individuals,[31] and this may be associated with generalized adenopathy throughout the body or localized to cervical region with associated adenotonsillar hypertrophy.

Chronic obstructive sialadenitis is commonly associated with chronic inflammation and obstruction of the gland. Patients often experience repeated episodes of acute painful gland swelling. The most common causes of chronic obstructive sialadenitis are salivary stones, mucous plugs, ductal stenosis, and foreign bodies.[31]

Salivary stones are thought to be the most common cause of chronic obstructive sialadenitis, although in the pediatric population this is still regarded as quite rare, accounting for less than 5% of reported cases.[31] Approximately 80% to 90% are found in the submandibular gland[31]; this is likely due to the mucinous nature of saliva produced by the submandibular gland. Ductal anatomy also plays a role because it requires saliva to flow against gravity.[31] Pediatric salivary stones are smaller, more distal in location, and present with a shorter duration of symptoms.[5,31]

Noninfectious

Sjögren syndrome is a chronic inflammatory autoimmune disease of the salivary and lacrimal glands along with many extraglandular manifestations.[33] This syndrome is considered to be comparatively rare in children, has an uncertain prognosis, and lacks standardized criteria. The pathogenesis is becoming more clearly understood, including the roles of T and B lymphocytes, autoantibodies, interferons, and glandular epithelial cells.[33] Means and colleagues[34] revealed an average of 4-year delay in the diagnosis from onset of symptoms, likely reflecting the difficulty in establishing the disease in children. Acute inflammatory symptoms of the parotid glands have been reported as the initial presenting symptom in children.[31,34] The gold standard for diagnosis is minor salivary gland biopsy. Immunologic testing should include antinuclear antibodies, and anti-double-stranded deoxyribonucleic acid antibodies for systemic lupus erythematosus and SS-A/anti-Ro (75%+), SS-B/anti-La antibodies (65%+) (O) for Sjögren syndrome. Vitali and colleagues[35] proposed classification criteria to include clinical symptoms of oral, ocular, and other mucosal inflammation with systemic inflammatory conditions as well as positive inflammatory and immune studies.[36]

No specific childhood Sjögren therapy or pathophysiology studies have been conducted. Sjögren treatment is largely symptomatic, aimed at improving or replacing exocrine gland function, and includes the use of sialogogues, artificial tears, and possible systemic therapies such as rituximab, a B-cell-depleting antibody, which has shown benefit in global Sjogren's disease.[33] Patients with Sjögren syndrome are known to be at serious risk for associated conditions with a 16-fold increased risk of non-Hodgkin lymphoma, permanent dental and ocular damage, gastrointestinal disorders, and pulmonary, renal, and liver disease, underscoring the need for high index of suspicion for early diagnosis and treatment.[34] Childhood Sjögren syndrome is a poorly defined and underdiagnosed condition. Efforts to define and evaluate new therapeutic modalities are ongoing. Additional studies are needed to establish preliminary childhood Sjögren classification criteria.

Juvenile Recurrent Parotitis

JRP is the second most common salivary disease involving children in the world after mumps and is the most reported cause of recurrent pediatric sialadenitis in the United States.[31,37] JRP is characterized as recurrent episodes of inflammation of the parotid gland. Symptoms include jaw swelling, pain, difficulty swallowing, and malaise. A clear cause is unknown, but a variety of factors are thought to include genetic, immune function, dehydration, congenital, allergy, ductal abnormalities, and/or obstruction.[31] Maynard[38] proposed that a low salivary flow caused by dehydration results in low-grade inflammation of the gland and duct epithelium. This inflammation then results in distortion and stricture of the distal duct and metaplasia of the ductal epithelium. These changes, along with a further reduction in salivary flow rate, predispose the gland to recurrent inflammation.

On examination, the gland is swollen, tender, and may have ductal mucopurulent discharge on gland compression. Most cases are unilateral: when bilateral cases occur, one side is usually dominant. The true incidence is unknown, and most reports are case series. Pediatric disease may have a male predominance, and age distribution is biphasic, typically between ages 2 and 6 years and again at the start of puberty.[31] The natural history is recurrence. Most investigators agree that this a self-limited disease that resolves sometime after puberty, although rare cases have extended into adulthood leading to a progressive loss of parenchymal function.[31,39] When studying JRP, a major concern is the lack of a shared definition of the disease. A review by Garavello and colleagues[40] did not arrive at any definitive conclusions for the treatment of JRP. The evidence was weak and difficult to interpret because of a scarcity of randomized controlled trials, the heterogeneity of definitions used, and high rate of spontaneous resolution. The study does propose diagnostic criteria for JRP (**Box 2**).[40]

The diagnosis of JRP is made clinically and with the exclusion of other diseases. Systemic diseases such as Sjögren and sarcoidosis should also be considered, and a referral to a pediatric rheumatologist may be considered. Symptoms typically last 4 to 7 days, and attacks occur every 3 to 4 months up to 10 times per year. Most consider JRP as self-limiting, and autoantibodies are usually absent. Early recognition of JRP and treatment are of utmost importance. Initial treatment aims to relieve symptoms and prevent further damage to gland parenchyma including nonsteroidal anti-

---

Box 2
Suggested criteria for the diagnosis of juvenile recurrent parotitis

Inclusion criteria
  Age less than 16 years
  Recurrent unilateral or bilateral parotid swelling
  At least 2 episodes in the last 6 months

Exclusion criteria
  Obstructive lesions
  Dental malocclusion
  Sjögren syndrome
  Congenital IgA immunodeficiency

---

inflammatory drugs, corticosteroids and antibiotics, warm compresses, hydration, and sialagogues.[40] Each attack may further tissue destruction and function of the gland.

Diagnostic Imaging Modalities

Various imaging modalities are available to assist in patient care. Imaging is more commonly used in the chronic setting but may aid in further investigation of acute complications.

High-resolution ultrasonography is the first-line imaging modality for the evaluation of the salivary glands[41]; it is easy to perform, requires minimal instrumentation, and eliminates exposure to radiation. Ultrasonography can assess gland/mass size, distinguish between solid and cystic masses, and evaluate ductal dilation as well as guide biopsy/aspiration.[5,31] The normal salivary gland is homogeneous in echotexture and hyperechogenic relative to adjacent musculature.[5] Features suggestive of chronic JRP include multiple hypoechoic lesions representing ductal ectasia, heterogeneous echogenicity, and sialectasis. Intraglandular lymph nodes and microcalcifications may also be present. Disadvantages of ultrasonography include its lower limit in stone detection of 2 mm, which may cause significant obstruction in the pediatric gland, and variable expertise of technician.

Computed tomography (CT) is particular helpful in evaluating air or microcalcifications as well as deeper structures.[5] CT is not operator dependent but is associated with ionizing radiation. CT can be useful for surgical planning, detailed abscess information, and recurrent infections that fail to demonstrate pathologic condition on ultrasonography.[31] MRI affords excellent soft tissue information and may aid in surgical planning as well.[5]

Management of Sialadenitis

The treatment of sialadenitis is usually conservative and directed toward cause. Viral infections are treated supportively with hydration, head elevation, gland massage, and sialagogues to stimulate salivary flow.[31] Bacterial diseases are treated with appropriate antibiotics covering aerobic and anaerobic pathogens.[42] Stones causing acute symptoms are managed conservatively initially with future plans for stone removal. Acute infection is, in general, contraindicated to surgical intervention due to risk of permanent injury and disease exacerbation.

Recurrent sialadenitis of the submandibular gland and JRP are treatment challenges. Acute management aims to relieve the symptoms and to limit parenchymal damage. Antibiotics and steroids are often favored as analgesics, sialagogues, hydration, massage, and warm compresses. Long-term management goals are aimed at reducing the frequency and severity of acute exacerbations. There is little evidence that conservative measures reduce the frequency of attacks. Traditional surgical management has included, gland excision, duct ligation, and tympanic neurectomy. Complications can be substantial and outcomes variable.

Long-term management of salivary stones has evolved over the last several decades from gland removal to preservation. Fluoroscopically guided stone retrieval and balloon dilation in the interventional radiology suite has been reported with some success but includes radiation exposure. Lithotripsy provides shock wave to achieve stone destruction leading to smaller pieces of the stone, which can then be excreted, and success in the pediatric population has been reported.[43]

Gland preservation is the paradigm shift in the management of chronic sialadenitis and sialolithiasis that encourages use of sialendoscopy. First reported by Katz[44] and more than 20 years ago, sialendoscopy has become the leading diagnostic technique and intervention for pediatric chronic/recurrent sialadenitis.[43] The advancements of using small, semirigid scopes with working channels have expanded the diagnostic and therapeutic possibilities in the pediatric population. Endoscopic visualization can help identify specific pathologic condition. Common findings of chronic sialadenitis include white ductal mucosal appearance indicating chronic inflammation, stenosis, mucous plug/debris, and stones (Fig. 2). Sialendoscopy has been reported to have a better sensitivity in diagnosing stones in children than CT, ultrasonography, and MRI.[45]

There are multiple semirigid endoscopes available, each with an irrigating channel and ranging in external diameter from 0.89 mm (diagnostic only) to 2.3 mm (with working channels) and with resolution between 6000 and 10,000 pixels. Saline (sodium chloride 0.9%) is used for irrigation and to dilate and visualize the ducts. The most commonly used scopes for therapeutic intervention in the pediatric population are the 1.1- and/or 1.3-mm scopes with working ports allowing for introduction of pharmacologic agents such as topical antibiotics and steroids, specialized wire baskets for stone extraction, laser fibers and drills for stone fulguration, and balloon dilators (Fig. 3).

Posttreatment may include antibiotics, steroid, and analgesic medication; it is regarded as an effective tool for evaluating and treating salivary pathology and allows the avoidance of the need for more invasive treatments such as sialoadenectomy, duct ligation, and tympanic neurectomy.[31]

This approach also allows for simultaneous intervention including ductal dilation, lavage, stone retrieval, and steroid application. Corticosteroid and/or antibiotic application is an accepted practice, although no formal studies have investigated the

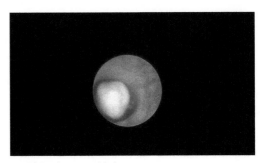

Fig. 2. Salivary stone within the parotid duct.

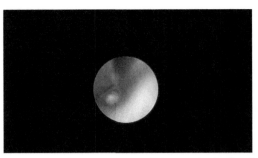

Fig. 3. View from a semirigid endoscope using utilizing a wire basket for stone extraction.

outcome of this technique.[31,46] Although the efficacy of sialendoscopy alone is well reported in up to 93% of patients with improvement or resolution of recurrent disease, combined procedures may be required with similar or improved success.[37,40] Small stones (2 to 3 mm) can be removed with wire baskets, whereas larger ones can be fragmented before removal. Additional techniques may be required for larger stones. This procedure generally requires general anesthesia and is rarely associated with complications. Results have shown gland and function preservation in more than 90% of patients.[47]

Analysis of the treatment of JRP suggests that sialendoscopy is safe, effective, and allows for gland preservation with functional gland recovery.[31,39,43,48,49] Most available evidence for the treatment of JRP has been focused on sialendoscopy including studies involving injecting various agents into the duct with reported added benefits.[40] Sialendoscopy is thought to improve JRP by washing out the intraductal debris and by dilating the stenotic duct.[39] There are, however, no randomized trials or agreed-upon protocols. Recurrence rate of up to 25.8% was noted in those treated with sialendoscopy.[40] It is important to consider that the procedure comes at added expense, requires experienced surgeons, and can cause discomfort and complications. Some studies have shown equal results with minimal to no intervention.[40] A review by Schwartz and colleagues[39] revealed that the endoscopic approach was most often used for the parotid gland (83%) followed by the submandibular gland (14.7%), which was not surprising because JRP was the most common diagnosis (68.9%) followed by sialolithiasis(14.5%). Recurrences occurred in 14.5% of pooled patients with JRP being the most common indication and ductal perforation being the most common complication.[31] Risks of sialendoscopy vary from 2% to 25%.[31] Complications are listed in **Box 3**.

To date, studies evaluating the treatment of JRP are limited by small patient populations, retrospective designs, and lack of control groups. Although sialendoscopy may be the key to better understand, diagnose, and treat JRP, future needs include large, long-term randomized trials to accurately determine the rate of disease's spontaneous resolutions and the best method of treatment.

SALIVARY GLAND NEOPLASMS

Salivary gland tumors are exceeding rare in the pediatric population. Neoplastic masses in children account for less than 5% of all benign and malignant tumors of the parotid gland occurring in patients younger than 16 years.[5,50] The age of the patient often aids in the diagnosis with vascular lesions presenting at birth or within a child's first year.[51] Solid tumors are more often encountered in older children.[52] Unlike

Box 3
Complications of sialendoscopy
Gland swelling
Ductal perforation
Delayed ductal stenosis
Ranula formation
Airway obstruction from excessive irrigation
Recurrence of obstruction
Failure to remove stone and/or remnants
Injury to ductal papilla
Ductal avulsion, necessitating gland removal

inflammatory disease with a more rapid onset and associated tenderness, neoplastic diseases have a more insidious course.[53] Persistent firm and nontender lesion should raise suspicion and require investigation with imaging and likely fine-needle aspiration. Large reviews of salivary gland lesions reveal just more than 4% occurring in children and 40% of these lesions were considered tumors.[54] Most studies report a higher incidence in malignancy in salivary tumors for children compared with adults, with the most common epithelial tumors being mucoepidermoid carcinoma and pleomorphic adenoma (PA) generally equal in frequency.[32,55] Pediatric salivary tumors have a heavy parotid dominance with the incidence of malignant tumors decreasing from parotid to submandibular to the sublingual glands, opposite to the tendency in adults.[50] Compared with adults, mesenchymal tumors are more common than epithelial tumors, of which hemangiomas are the most frequent.[50] The differential for salivary masses is included in **Box 4**.

Benign Epithelial Tumors

Pleomorphic adenoma

PAs account for half of all epithelial tumors of the salivary glands and more than 90% of benign salivary gland epithelial tumors.[51] Most occur in the parotid gland (62%), followed by the submandibular gland (26%) with a female to male ratio of 1.4:1.[51] Symptoms include slow-growing, firm, painless mass of approximately 1 year duration. On CT, small calcifications can be seen, and on MRI they are very bright on T2-weighted images. Histologic features include epithelial/myoepithelial cells and a myxochondroid matrix.[54] Treatment is surgical removal with superficial or total parotidectomy depending on tumor location, leading to 95% local control of disease.[55] Simple enucleation of the lesion is not advised with a recurrence rate of more than 40% associated with the treatment.[54] PAs do possess the potential for malignant degeneration. The estimated risk is about 6% and seems to be associated with length of tumor presence. These carcinoma ex-PAs are exceeding rare in children. Given the long life expectancy, and a known recurrence rate of up to 30 years after the initial resection, there is an increased risk of recurrence in children, resulting in need for long-term follow-up.[51]

Benign Mesenchymal Tumors

Hemangioma

Hemangiomas account for 90% of all salivary gland tumors in children younger than 1 year with about 30% present at birth.[51] In some series they account for up to half

---

Box 4
Differential diagnoses for a salivary mass

Nonneoplastic
    Congenital: first branchial arch anomalies
    Inflammatory/infectious: reactive intraglandular lymph node, glandular abscess
    Cystic disease: ranula, mucocele

Neoplastic benign disease
    Epithelial: pleomorphic adenoma
    Mesenchymal: hemangioma, vascular malformation, neurofibroma

Neoplastic malignant disease
    Epithelial: mucoepidermoid carcinoma, acinic cell carcinoma, adenoid cystic carcinoma, adenocarcinoma
    Mesenchymal: rhabdomyosarcoma, liposarcoma
    Lymphoma

---

of all salivary gland tumors. Hemangiomas undergo a distinct pattern of development, proliferating rapidly in the first months of life; this is generally followed by a second growth spurt in the fourth to sixth months of life, and then they begin to slowly involute, often completely by the first decade. Approximately 80% to 90% arise in the parotid gland with the rest mainly in the submandibular glands.[5,51]

Hemangiomas are soft, unilateral masses with or without bluish discoloration of the skin; they may present as focal masses centered in the parotid space or as segmental lesion involving the parotid gland as well as adjacent soft tissue in the V3 trigeminal nerve distribution. Those of the segmental variety may be accompanied by abnormalities of the PHACES association (posterior fossa malformation, carotid and cerebral arterial anomalies, cardiac defects, aortic coarctation, eye abnormalities, and sternal or other ventral defects).[5] Segmental lesions are also more likely to be associated with medical complications including airway compromise, skin ulceration, and soft tissue destruction.[5]

Imaging modalities show a lobulated, solid hypervascular mass. Histologically, they are unencapsulated aggregates of capillaries with endothelial cells separated by scant connective tissue. On MRI, they are generally T1 isointense and T2 hyperintense compared with muscle. Treatment may not be required unless it is complicated by skin ulceration, infection, or airway compression. Management may include consideration of the use of propranolol.[56,57] The proposed mechanism of action includes rapid vasoconstriction of the lesion. Inhibition of angiogenesis by downregulation of proangiogenic growth factors, vascular endothelial growth factor, basic fibroblast growth factor, and matric metalloproteinases 2 and 9 seems to correspond with growth arrest; it may hasten apoptosis of the endothelial cells as well. Surgical therapy, gland removal, is reserved for those not responding to medical therapy with associated cosmetic or obstructive complications.

Lymphatic malformations

Lymphatic malformations (LMs) are congenital anomalies of the lymphatic system with 90% detected by age 2 years.[51] LMs are the second most common mesenchymal tumor.[32] LMs often present suddenly as palpable mass related to a recent infection or intralesional hemorrhage. On MRI LMs are well-circumscribed, multicystic masses predominantly bright on T2-weighted images. Phleboliths appear as signal voids on MRI and are the hallmark of low-flow malformation. On ultrasonography, macrocystic lesions are compressible, nonvascular anechoic lesions that are most commonly unilocular with thin septae.[5] Microcystic lesions are hyperechoic and more poorly defined.[5]

Histologically, LMs are a complex of multiple cysts lined with lymphatic vascular endothelium. Unlike hemangiomas of infancy, LMs do not undergo spontaneous regression. Treatment options included sclerotherapy with OK-432, doxycycline, or ethanol for macrocystic lesions, surgery, or combination.

Malignant Epithelial Tumors

Malignancies of the salivary glands in children are extremely rare, with an annual estimated incidence of 0.08 per 100,000.[58] Literature reviews conclude that pediatric cases of salivary cancer represent less than 5% of all salivary malignancies, and the vast majority represents epithelial neoplasms.[58] Overall, salivary gland malignancies in children comprise only 8% to 10% of all pediatric head and neck cancers.[3] Most information regarding this disease is acquired from retrospective studies at tertiary oncologic institutions. Approximately 50% of major salivary gland tumors in children are malignant, which is twice the proportion reported for adults.[52] The most common anatomic site for malignant salivary gland tumors is the parotid gland (80%), followed by minor salivary glands and submandibular glands.[51] Children have a higher percentage (88%) of well-differentiated tumors than adults, which carries an overall better prognosis.[59] Most malignant salivary gland tumors occur in older children/adolescents with an average age of presentation of 13 years. Benign tumors tend to present a bit later at age 15 years, and sex distribution seems to be equal. Cancers presenting at less than age 10 years are more likely to be high grade and are associated with a poorer prognosis.[3] The cause is largely unknown with some studies linking exposure to Epstein-Barr virus and others noting prior exposure to radiation and chemotherapy increasing the risk of development.[3,58] Mucoepidermoid carcinoma is the most common malignant tumor (60%), followed by acinic cell carcinoma (11%), adenocarcinoma (10%), and adenoid cystic carcinoma (9%).[51]

Salivary neoplasms present as a firm mass and have usually been present for 8 to 12 months; they are often asymptomatic, although pain is occasionally present most commonly with adenoid cystic carcinoma. The mass may be fixated to surrounding tissue, and rarely the facial nerve may be weak. Enlarged lymph nodes are rarely present in children (3.5%).[51]

Ultrasonography is helpful in distinguishing solid from cystic masses and in approximating tumor size. MRI allows for more detailed soft tissue information but often requires sedation for children.[34] CT is useful in assessing the size of the lesion, defining bone involvement, and demonstrating lymph node metastases. However, it does expose the patient to ionizing radiation and may require sedation. Fine-needle aspiration cytology is a helpful tool and may require sedation; its accuracy has been reported to be quite variable and as low as 33%.[4]

Treatment of salivary gland tumors is complete surgical removal with adequate margins.[60] For submandibular disease, complete gland removal is recommended. In general, the same is true for the parotid gland, especially for aggressive tumors with high risk of recurrence. Definitive surgery allows for excellent local control of up to 97%.[3,60] Surgery of the parotid gland does incur a risk of injury to the facial nerve with resulting temporary or permanent paresis or paralysis. Use of regional lymph node dissection, perioperative radiation therapy, and chemotherapy is individualized and best determined by an oncological team. Overall prognosis remains quite favorable, and survival rates range from 80% to 95%, especially for those diagnosed at an early stage and whose tumors are low grade and completely resected.[3,61]

Malignant Mesenchymal Tumors

Rhabdomyosarcoma

Rhabdomyosarcomas of the salivary glands are exceedingly uncommon with a suspected incidence of 2% to 3% of salivary malignancies in children[54]; they are the most common pediatric soft tissue sarcoma, and 40% occur in the head and neck.[58] Rhabdomyosarcomas present as swelling that often rapidly increases in size. About 70% occur between age 1 and 9 years[58]; they have a much shorter duration of symptoms (5 weeks) with pain and facial weakness more commonly seen. Any suspicion for this tumor should lead to obtaining an MRI with earlier detection improving chances for a complete resection. Unfortunately, most present with locally invasive or metastatic disease making complete resection less likely and necessitating the need for adjuvant chemotherapy and radiation. Prognosis is not well determined, but one larger series reported a 5-year survival rate of 84%.[51] Multicenter longitudinal studies are needed to evaluate the role of adjuvant therapies with goals of improving local control and preventing distant metastasis.

DISCLOSURE

The authors have nothing to disclose.

REFERENCES

1. Aro K, Leivo I, Mäkitie A. Management of salivary gland malignancies in the pediatric population. Curr Opin Otolaryngol Head Neck Surg 2014;22(2):116–20.
2. Krolls SO, Trodahl JN, Boyers RC. Salivary gland lesions in children. A survey of 430 cases. Cancer 1972;30(2):459–69.
3. Yoshida EJ, García J, Eisele DW, et al. Salivary gland malignancies in children. Int J Pediatr Otorhinolaryngol 2014;78(2):174–8.
4. Védrine PO, Coffinet L, Temam S, et al. Mucoepidermoid carcinoma of salivary glands in the pediatric age group: 18 clinical cases, including 11 second malignant neoplasms. Head Neck 2006;28(9):827–33.
5. Friedman E, Patiño MO, Udayasankar UK. Imaging of Pediatric Salivary Glands. Neuroimaging Clin N Am 2018;28(2):209–26.
6. Som PM, Miletech I. The Embryology of the Salivary Glands: An Update. Neurographics 2015;5(4):167–77.
7. Matsuo R. Role of saliva in the maintenance of taste sensitivity. Crit Rev Oral Biol Med 2000;11(2):216–29.
8. Fox PC, Eversole LR. Diseases of the salivary glands. In: Silverman S, Eversole LR, Truelove EL, editors. Essentials of oral medicine. Hamilton, Ontario, Canada: BC Decker; 2002. p. 260–76.
9. Tabak LA, Levine MJ, Mandel ID, et al. Role of salivary mucins in the protection of the oral cavity. J Oral Pathol 1982;11(1):1–17.
10. Porte M, Chaléat-Valayer E, Patte K, et al. Relevance of intraglandular injections of Botulinum toxin for the treatment of sialorrhea in children with cerebral palsy: a review. Eur J Paediatr Neurol 2014;18(6):649–57.
11. Hockstein NG, Samadi DS, Gendron K, et al. Sialorrhea: a management challenge. Am Fam Physician 2004;69(11):2628–34.
12. Pham Dang N, Picard M, Mondié JM, et al. Complete congenital agenesis of all major salivary glands: a case report and review of the literature. Oral Surg Oral Med Oral Pathol Oral Radiol Endod 2010;110(4):e23–7.

13. Finn DG, Buchalter IH, Sarti E, et al. First branchial cleft cysts: clinical update. Laryngoscope 1987;97(2):136–40.
14. Pandit RT, Park AH. Management of pediatric ranula. Otolaryngol Head Neck Surg 2002;127(1):115–8.
15. Seo JH, Park JJ, Kim HY, et al. Surgical management of intraoral ranulas in children: an analysis of 17 pediatric cases. Int J Pediatr Otorhinolaryngol 2010;74(2): 202–5.
16. Jost WH, Bäumer T, Laskawi R, et al. Therapy of Sialorrhea with Botulinum Neurotoxin. Neurol Ther 2019;8(2):273–88.
17. Sousa S, Rocha M, Patrão F, et al. Submandibular duct transposition for drooling in children: A Casuistic review and evaluation of grade of satisfaction. Int J Pediatr Otorhinolaryngol 2018;113:58–61.
18. Hughes A, Choi S. Does intraglandular injection of botulinum toxin improve pediatric sialorrhea? Laryngoscope 2018;128(7):1513–4.
19. Jablenska L, Trinidade A, Meranagri V, et al. Salivary gland pathology in the paediatric population: implications for management and presentation of a rare case. J Laryngol Otol 2014;128(1):104–6.
20. Leung AK, Kao CP. Drooling in children. Paediatr Child Health 1999;4(6):406–11.
21. Little SA, Kubba H, Hussain SS. An evidence-based approach to the child who drools saliva. Clin Otolaryngol 2009;34(3):236–9.
22. Jongerius PH, Rotteveel JJ, van den Hoogen F, et al. Botulinum toxin A: a new option for treatment of drooling in children with cerebral palsy. Presentation of a case series. Eur J Pediatr 2001;160(8):509–12.
23. Lawrence R, Bateman N. Surgical Management of the Drooling Child. Curr Otorhinolaryngol Rep 2018;6(1):99–106.
24. Alvarenga A, Campos M, Dias M, et al. BOTOX-A injection of salivary glands for drooling. J Pediatr Surg 2017;52(8):1283–6.
25. Rodwell K, Edwards P, Ware RS, et al. Salivary gland botulinum toxin injections for drooling in children with cerebral palsy and neurodevelopmental disability: a systematic review. Dev Med Child Neurol 2012;54(11):977–87.
26. El-Hakim H, Richards S, Thevasagayam MS. Major salivary duct clipping for control problems in developmentally challenged children. Arch Otolaryngol Head Neck Surg 2008;134(5):470–4.
27. Kok SE, van der Burg JJ, van Hulst K, et al. The impact of submandibular duct relocation on drooling and the well-being of children with neurodevelopmental disabilities. Int J Pediatr Otorhinolaryngol 2016;88:173–8.
28. Delsing CP, Cillessen E, Scheffer A, et al. Bilateral submandibular gland excision for drooling: Our experience in twenty-six children and adolescents. Clin Otolaryngol 2015;40(3):285–90.
29. Stern Y, Feinmesser R, Collins M, et al. Bilateral submandibular gland excision with parotid duct ligation for treatment of sialorrhea in children: long-term results. Arch Otolaryngol Head Neck Surg 2002;128(7):801–3.
30. Reed J, Mans CK, Brietzke SE. Surgical management of drooling: a meta-analysis. Arch Otolaryngol Head Neck Surg 2009;135(9):924–31.
31. Francis CL, Larsen CG. Pediatric sialadenitis. Otolaryngol Clin North Am 2014; 47(5):763–78.
32. Carlson ER, Ord RA. Benign Pediatric Salivary Gland Lesions. Oral Maxillofac Surg Clin N Am 2016;28(1):67–81.
33. Lieberman SM. Childhood Sjögren syndrome: insights from adults and animal models. Curr Opin Rheumatol 2013;25(5):651–7.

34. Means C, Aldape MA, King E. Pediatric primary Sjögren syndrome presenting with bilateral ranulas: A case report and systematic review of the literature. Int J Pediatr Otorhinolaryngol 2017;101:11–9.
35. Vitali C, Bombardieri S, Jonsson R, et al. Classification criteria for Sjögren's syndrome: a revised version of the European criteria proposed by the American-European Consensus Group. Ann Rheum Dis 2002;61(6):554–8.
36. Shiboski SC, Shiboski CH, Criswell L, et al. American College of Rheumatology classification criteria for Sjögren's syndrome: a data-driven, expert consensus approach in the Sjögren's International Collaborative Clinical Alliance cohort. Arthritis Care Res (Hoboken) 2012;64(4):475–87.
37. Wood J, Toll EC, Hall F, et al. Juvenile recurrent parotitis: Review and proposed management algorithm. Int J Pediatr Otorhinolaryngol 2021;142:110617.
38. Maynard JD. Recurrent parotid enlargement. Br J Surg 1965;52(10):784–9.
39. Schwarz Y, Bezdjian A, Daniel SJ. Sialendoscopy in treating pediatric salivary gland disorders: a systematic review. Eur Arch Otorhinolaryngol 2018;275(2):347–56.
40. Garavello W, Redaelli M, Galluzzi F, et al. Juvenile recurrent parotitis: A systematic review of treatment studies. Int J Pediatr Otorhinolaryngol 2018;112:151–7.
41. Sodhi KS, Bartlett M, Prabhu NK. Role of high resolution ultrasound in parotid lesions in children. Int J Pediatr Otorhinolaryngol 2011;75(11):1353–8.
42. Brook I. Diagnosis and management of parotitis. Arch Otolaryngol Head Neck Surg 1992;118(5):469–71.
43. Fritsch MH. Sialendoscopy and lithotripsy: literature review. Otolaryngol Clin North Am 2009;42(6).
44. Katz P. Nouvelle thérapeutique des lithiases salivaires [New treatment method for salivary lithiasis]. Rev Laryngol Otol Rhinol (Bord) 1993;114(5):379–82.
45. Martins-Carvalho C, Plouin-Gaudon I, Quenin S, et al. Pediatric sialendoscopy: a 5-year experience at a single institution. Arch Otolaryngol Head Neck Surg 2010;136(1):33–6.
46. Papadopoulou-Alataki E, Dogantzis P, Chatziavramidis A, et al. Juvenile Recurrent Parotitis: The Role of Sialendoscopy. Int J Inflam 2019;2019:7278907.
47. Faure F, Querin S, Dulguerov P, et al. Pediatric salivary gland obstructive swelling: sialendoscopic approach. Laryngoscope 2007;117(8):1364–7.
48. Bruch JM, Setlur J. Pediatric sialendoscopy. Adv Otorhinolaryngol 2012;73:149–52.
49. Canzi P, Occhini A, Pagella F, et al. Sialendoscopy in juvenile recurrent parotitis: a review of the literature. Acta Otorhinolaryngol Ital 2013;33(6):367–73.
50. Luna MA, Batsakis JG, el-Naggar AK. Salivary gland tumors in children. Ann Otol Rhinol Laryngol 1991;100(10):869–71.
51. Lennon P, Silvera VM, Perez-Atayde A, et al. Disorders and tumors of the salivary glands in children. Otolaryngol Clin North Am 2015;48(1):153–73.
52. da Cruz Perez DE, Pires FR, Alves FA, et al. Salivary gland tumors in children and adolescents: a clinicopathologic and immunohistochemical study of fifty-three cases. Int J Pediatr Otorhinolaryngol 2004;68(7):895–902.
53. Koch BL, Myer CM 3rd. Presentation and diagnosis of unilateral maxillary swelling in children. Am J Otolaryngol 1999;20(2):106–29.
54. Krolls SO, Boyers RC. Mixed tumors of salivary glands. Long-term Follow-up Cancer 1972;30(1):276–81.
55. Leverstein H, van der Wal JE, Tiwari RM, et al. Surgical management of 246 previously untreated pleomorphic adenomas of the parotid gland. Br J Surg 1997;84(3):399–403.

56. Léauté-Labrèze C, Dumas de la Roque E, Hubiche T, et al. Propranolol for severe hemangiomas of infancy. N Engl J Med 2008;358(24):2649–51.

57. Oosthuizen JC, Burns P, Russell JD. Lymphatic malformations: a proposed management algorithm. Int J Pediatr Otorhinolaryngol 2010;74(4):398–403.

58. Ord RA, Carlson ER. Pediatric Salivary Gland Malignancies. Oral Maxillofac Surg Clin N Am 2016;28(1):83–9.

59. Sultan I, Rodriguez-Galindo C, Al-Sharabati S, et al. Salivary gland carcinomas in children and adolescents: a population-based study, with comparison to adult cases. Head Neck 2011;33(10):1476–81.

60. Rahbar R, Grimmer JF, Vargas SO, et al. Mucoepidermoid carcinoma of the parotid gland in children: A 10-year experience. Arch Otolaryngol Head Neck Surg 2006;132(4):375–80.

61. Louredo BVR, Santos-Silva AR, Vargas PA, et al. Clinicopathological analysis and survival outcomes of primary salivary gland tumors in pediatric patients: A systematic review. J Oral Pathol Med 2021;50(5):435–43.

Otolaryngologic Disease in Down syndrome

Marisa A. Earley, MD*, Erica T. Sher, MD, Tess L. Hill, MD

KEYWORDS

- Otolaryngology • Down syndrome • Trisomy 21 • Obstructive sleep apnea
- Dysphagia • Upper airway obstruction • Hearing loss

KEY POINTS

- Obstructive sleep apnea (OSA) is less likely to be adequately treated by adenotonsillectomy in patients with Down syndrome (DS). Primary drug-induced sleep endoscopy (DISE) and the need for further surgery or positive airway pressure (PAP) treatment should be considered.
- Feeding difficulty is multifactorial and early involvement of SLP is critical even if surgery is to be considered.
- Craniofacial morphology, hypotonia, and upper and lower airway abnormalities contribute to high incidence of airway obstruction, resulting in difficulties with breathing, sleeping, and feeding.
- Many patients with DS will have some hearing loss, most commonly conductive in nature, secondary to underlying Eustachian tube dysfunction and middle ear effusions.
- Patients with DS have a higher risk of anesthetic complications due to congenital cardiac disease, pulmonary disease, and airway abnormalities. It is, therefore, important to have well-trained anesthesiologists and adequate postoperative monitoring.

INTRODUCTION

As the most common chromosomal abnormality in humans with an annual incidence of 1 in every 700 to 800 births,[1] Down syndrome (DS) is a condition that the otolaryngologist will undoubtedly encounter. In 2011, the Committee on Genetics released health supervision recommendations for children with DS.[2] **Table 1** reviews the most encountered medical problems in patients with DS. A significant number of these problems are managed by the otolaryngologist (hearing problems, obstructive sleep apnea (OSA), otitis media, thyroid disease) or impact care delivered by the otolaryngologist (congenital heart disease (CHD), hypotonia, seizures, hematologic problems, atlanto-axial instability, autism). In a review of national data, Patel and colleagues

UT Health San Antonio, 7703 Floyd Curl Drive MC 7777, San Antonio, TX 78229, USA
* Corresponding author.
E-mail address: earleyma@uthscsa.edu

Pediatr Clin N Am 69 (2022) 381–401
https://doi.org/10.1016/j.pcl.2022.01.005
0031-3955/22/© 2022 Elsevier Inc. All rights reserved.

Table 1
Common medical problems in pediatric patients with Down syndrome.

Condition	%
Hearing problems	75
Vision problems	60
Cataracts	15
Refractive errors	50
Obstructive sleep apnea	50-75
Otitis media	50-70
Congenital heart disease	40-50
Hypodontia and delayed dental eruption	23
Gastrointestinal atresias	12
Thyroid disease	4-18
Seizures	1-13
Hematologic problems	
Anemia	3
Iron deficiency	10
Transient myeloproliferative disorder	10
Leukemia	1
Celiac disease	5
Atlanto-axial instability	1-2
Autism	1
Hirschsprung disease	<1

Data from Bull MJ; Committee on Genetics. Health supervision for children with Down syndrome [published correction appears in Pediatrics. 2011 Dec;128(6):1212]. Pediatrics. 2011;128(2):393-406. https://doi.org/10.1542/peds.2011-1605 (permission pending)

discovered that patients with DS are significantly over-represented in various pediatric otolaryngologic procedures including tracheostomy, endoscopy, laryngoscopy, tracheoplasty, myringoplasty, tympanoplasty with mastoidectomy, and tympanoplasty without mastoidectomy.[3] They also found that patients with DS were under-represented in various categories as well such as abscess, palatoplasty, excision of congenital neck cyst and cochlear implantation.[3] Upper airway obstruction and otologic disorders are exceedingly common in patients with DS and are often managed by an otolaryngologist.[3–7] Also of great importance to the otolaryngologist is the awareness that CHD occurs in 40% of children with DS.[8] Further, we will review various anesthetic and wound healing considerations in this patient population that impact delivery of care, particularly surgical intervention. This article will serve to review otolaryngologic manifestations in DS as well as perioperative special considerations.

BREATHING, SLEEPING, AND SWALLOWING
Anatomic Considerations

The craniofacial morphology in patients with DS includes shorter anterior and posterior cranial base length, smaller maxillary length, greater tendency for class 3 occlusion, brachyfacial pattern (open mouth and anterior open bite deformity), and reduced facial height.[9,10] Yet despite these unique facial features, a recent study demonstrated that patients with DS quantitatively resemble their siblings; this provides evidence of genetic impact on the resemblance between relatives even with the impact of the DS genotype on craniofacial morphology.[11]

Interestingly, the distinctive facial features in patients with DS (**Figs. 1** and **2**) likely do not solely have a causative effect on upper airway obstruction. This is based on the fact that 3D photogrammetric measurements could not distinguish between patients with DS that had or did not have OSA.[11] These morphologic changes in addition to other physiologic features result in upper airway obstruction, which is the most common reason for referral to the pediatric otolaryngologist.[3] Therefore, it is the internal airway anatomy with nasal and midface hypoplasia, pharyngeal narrowing, relative macroglossia, combined with hypotonia that contributes to upper airway obstruction, OSA, and dysphagia.

Prevalence of OSA in children with DS was 66% based on full night polysomnography in a study by Maris and colleagues and even in those patients with a negative history of OSA, the prevalence was still 54%.[12] This reinforces the need for polysomnography in this patient population, as history alone is an inadequate predictor of OSA. In infants with DS, 90% of infants who underwent a video-fluoroscopic swallow study (VFSS) had at least one element of oral dysphagia and 72% had at least one element of pharyngeal dysphagia.[13]

Evaluation

The otolaryngologist plays a critical role in the evaluation of patients with DS when it comes to abnormalities with breathing, sleeping, and swallowing (**Box 1**). The

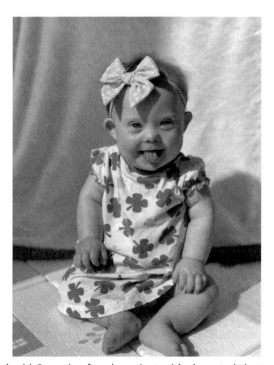

Fig. 1. Eight-month-old Caucasian female patient with characteristic craniofacial morphologic features seen in Down syndrome.

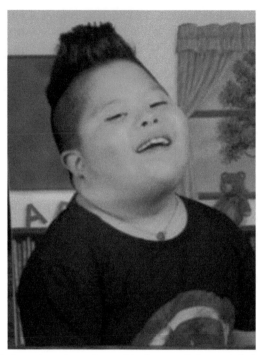

Fig. 2. Six-year-old Hispanic male patient with characteristic craniofacial morphologic features seen in Down syndrome.

American Academy of Pediatrics (AAP) has multiple recommendations related to otolaryngologic manifestations in patients with DS.[2] The AAP recommends in the earliest period (birth to 1 month of life) children with DS should be assessed for stridor or noisy breathing due to the risk of laryngotracheal anomalies and/or feeding difficulty. Starting at birth, radiographic swallowing assessment is recommended if there is significant hypotonia, feeding difficulty (slow feeding, choking with feeds, recurrent or persistent respiratory symptoms), or failure to thrive. They also recommend having a laboratory based polysomnogram by the age of 4, as parents are not reliable in assessing for sleep apnea and home studies are also inaccurate.[2,7,14,15]

Hamilton and colleagues sought to determine the prevalence of airway problems in children with DS. In a retrospective review of 20 years of data with a true denominator for the number of children with DS in the specific region of Scotland, 16% of pediatric patients with DS underwent microlaryngoscopy and bronchoscopy (MLB) for airway symptoms. Eighty-four percent of these patients were found to have at least one airway diagnosis including tracheobronchomalacia, laryngeal cleft, laryngomalacia, tracheal compression, vocal cord paralysis, acquired tracheal stenosis, and symptomatic subglottic stenosis.[16] This represented 14% of the total pediatric DS population.

Full airway evaluation with combined bronchoscopy with pulmonary and otolaryngology is often able to be accomplished in the same day and same anesthetic. In one retrospective review, 96% of pediatric patients with DS undergoing both flexible bronchoscopy and MLB had at least 1 airway abnormality, 33% had 2%, and 46% had 3 or more abnormalities.[17] The most common findings (**Box 2**) were tracheomalacia, subglottic stenosis, pharyngomalacia, and laryngomalacia. Many studies recognize

---

Box 1
Modalities for evaluation of airway, feeding, and sleep in pediatric patients with Down syndrome

History and physical examination

Flexible fiberoptic transnasal laryngoscopy

Microlaryngoscopy and rigid bronchoscopy

Flexible bronchoscopy ± bronchoalveolar lavage

Instrumental Swallow Assessment (VFSS, MBS, FEES)

Laboratory-based polysomnogram

DISE ± intervention

Imaging

Abbreviations: VFSS, video-fluoroscopic swallow study; MBS, modified barium swallow; FEES, fiberoptic endoscopic evaluation of swallow; DISE, drug-induced sleep endoscopy.

---

the difficulty in knowing the true incidence of laryngomalacia in this patient population.[18,19] Diagnostic evaluation of the airway of a pediatric DS patient should involve a lower threshold for lower airway endoscopy, swallow studies, and imaging due to a much higher prevalence of lower airway problems.[20] Further, pediatric patients with DS have a higher incidence of silent aspiration and they often have more refractory respiratory tract infections and/or pulmonary hypertension, which can complicate the management of respiratory and airway disease.[21]

In a systematic review of tracheal anomalies associated with DS, tracheal anomalies occur more frequently and tracheal surgery (ie, tracheostomy and tracheoplasty) is performed more frequently in DS compared with nonsyndromic children. Complaints suggestive of airway obstruction such as stridor, dyspnea, and wheezing that is refractory to medical management should lead the otolaryngologist to perform diagnostic rigid tracheobronchoscopy.[22] In a study by De Lausnay and colleagues, congenital airway anomalies were seen in 71% of patients with DS compared with 32% of controls and combined anomalies were more frequent with DS. **Table 2** lists common laryngotracheal abnormalities in children with DS. Based on this high prevalence, lower airway endoscopy is recommended in addition to upper airway evaluation in patients with DS as this may influence decision making, particularly for patients with recurrent respiratory infections, chronic cough and noisy breathing.[20] In a classic study by Shott et al, MRI of the trachea of DS children without respiratory symptoms showed tracheal diameter 1.3 to 3.2 mm smaller compared with age-matched non-DS

Box 2
Common laryngotracheal abnormalities in pediatric Down syndrome patients.

Airway malacia (laryngo-, tracheo-, broncho-, or multilevel) Subglottic stenosis (congenital or acquired)
Complete tracheal ring
Tracheal bronchus
Tracheal compression by vascular structures
Tracheal web
Congenital or acquired tracheal stenosis

children. Therefore, they recommend using an endotracheal tube that is 0.5 to 1.5 mm smaller than recommendations based on age and to assess for an audible leak at 10 to 30 cm H_2O.[23] Of note, tracheal stenosis is highly correlated with confirmed CHD.[24]

Skotko and colleagues developed a predictive model of OSA in patients with DS using examination, history, lateral cephalogram, 3D photograph, and validated sleep questionnaires. They found that with simple procedures that can be collected at minimal cost, the proposed model could predict which patients with DS were unlikely to have moderate to severe OSA and thus may not need a diagnostic sleep study.[25] Many authors also support the use of drug-induced sleep endoscopy (DISE) in the evaluation of surgically naïve patients with DS and OSA.[26–28]

Therapeutic Options

Management of upper airway obstruction is highly variable depending on symptoms. Surgical intervention often mirrors the recommendations for nonsyndromic children; however, success rates are significantly lower and this must be discussed extensively with families and other treating health care providers to manage expectations. For example, if the evaluation reveals laryngomalacia, there is only a 62% to 66% success rate for supraglottoplasty compared with 95% success in non-DS children and 50% of patients with DS required additional airway surgery.[18,19] The vast majority of DS infants with laryngomalacia do demonstrate improved breathing, feeding and sleeping after supraglottoplasty.[18] Patients with DS and laryngomalacia also often have other causes of dysphagia that will require extensive therapy by a speech and language pathologist (SLP) both before and after surgical intervention.[13,18,29] In fact, swallowing

Table 2			
Recommendations for otolaryngologic evaluations or screenings in patients with Down syndrome			
Age	**Otolaryngologic Evaluations or Screenings**		
Birth to 1 mo	Screen for feeding difficulties Congenital hearing loss via NBHS (ABR) Screen for GERD Screen for noisy breathing Check laboratories for congenital hypothyroidism		
1 mo to 1 y	Confirm hearing screen results Ear examination by otolaryngologist every 3–6 mo until tympanic membrane can be visualized by pediatrician or tympanometry can be performed reliably Discuss symptoms of OSA		
1 y to 5 y	Test hearing every 6 mo until normal hearing levels are found bilaterally on ear specific evaluations Image for atlanto-axial instability in the symptomatic patient over age 3 Perform PSG to evaluate for OSA by age 4 y		
5 y to 13 y	Perform annual ear specific audiogram Measure TSH annually Discuss symptoms of OSA at every visit		
13 y to >21 y	Perform annual ear specific audiogram Measure TSH annually Discuss symptoms of OSA at every visit		

Abbreviations: NBHS, New Born Hearing Screen; ABR, Auditory Brainstem Response; GERD, Gastroesophageal Reflux Disease, OSA, obstructive sleep apnea; PSG, polysomnogram; TSH, Thyroid Stimulating Hormone

assessments in DS infants with dysphagia have been shown to change over time and often require more repeat testing as the child ages.[30] Tongue and lip strength are also significantly lower in children with DS, therefore, this should also be addressed by SLP.[31]

Rates of tracheostomy for pediatric DS population are three times higher than the general pediatric population. Additional, over half of the pediatric DS tracheostomy patients had a primary indication of airway obstruction, while patients with non-DS were more likely to have prematurity related cardiopulmonary respiratory failure as the indication for tracheostomy.[32]

Surgical management of OSA in patients with DS, similar to surgery for laryngomalacia, has the same first-line recommendation of adenotonsillectomy (AT) as the most commonly performed procedure in both patients with DS and non-DS; however, AT has significantly lower success rates in the DS population.[26–28,33–39] Cure rate with AT in patients with nonsyndromic is 60% to 80% while in patients with DS is less than 20%. After treatment with AT alone, up to 75% of patients with DS will need postoperative respiratory support while sleeping and only a 51% decrease in AHI can be.[33]

Despite poorer surgical outcomes, demographic, clinical factors and preoperative PSG data failed to predict persistent OSA and OSA severity after AT.[36] A large single-institution study demonstrated an overall morbidity rate of 32% from AT in DS children.[37] The most common morbidity was respiratory-related (54% of morbidity including recurrent desaturations, aspiration pneumonia or prolonged intubation), followed by poor PO intake (37%) and bleeding (18%). This study also demonstrated that 29% of patients with DS undergoing AT had a prolonged hospital stay. All of these factors are critical to consider when counseling parents and assessing health care resource utilization.[37]

Due to the poor cure rate for AT alone, there is increasing literature supporting primary DISE for surgically naïve patients with DS with OSA instead of reserving for use after failure of AT.[26–28,38,39] In the cohort study by Hyzer and colleagues assessing DISE findings in various groups, surgically naïve children with obesity and OSA had primarily tonsillar obstruction while DS children had higher rates of obstruction at the level of tonsils, tongue base and arytenoids compared with control patients.[28] Wootten and colleagues had a 92% parental satisfaction rate with DS patients' postoperative breathing after DISE directed surgical treatment.[38] DISE directed surgical intervention often involves addressing the tongue base and/or lingual tonsils in both DS and non-DS pediatric patients. **Fig. 3** demonstrates an algorithm for the management of OSA in children with DS based on severity. These interventions are effective in normal weight and overweight children with DS, but not in those with pre- or postoperative obesity. Therefore, authors strongly advise aggressive weight loss initiatives.[40,41] **Fig. 4** contains important consensus statements regarding pediatric DISE and **Fig. 5** contains pediatric DISE scoring template and representative photos.

An important factor to note is that many pediatric patients with DS will still require additional intervention after surgery due to persistent symptoms. **Fig. 6** demonstrates an algorithm for the management of residual OSA after AT. Studies demonstrate that though compliance with positive airway pressure (PAP) can be a difficulty, it is typically only difficult within the first year of initiating treatment and if parents and providers persist, many children will tolerate it.[42] Further, despite concern over pediatric DS patients' ability to tolerate PSG, a recent study demonstrated that 96% of patients tolerated PSG and 86% were able to sleep beyond 4 hours. PAP titration was tolerated in 83% of children with DS in this study.[43] If PAP is not tolerated, there is literature to support the use of high flow nasal cannula, though this must be studied further in this particular patient population.[42,44]

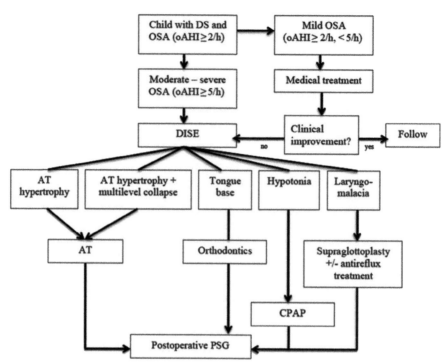

Fig. 3. Proposed algorithm for the management of obstructive sleep apnea in children with Down syndrome and obstructive sleep apnea based on polysomnography results. OSA, obstructive sleep apnea; oAHI, obstructive Apnea-Hypopnea Index; AT, adenotonsillectomy; CPAP, continuous positive airway pressure; PSG, polysomnogram. (*Data from* Maris M, Verhulst S, Saldien V, Van de Heyning P, Wojciechowski M, Boudewyns A. Drug-induced sedation endoscopy in surgically naive children with Down syndrome and obstructive sleep apnea. *Sleep Med.* 2016;24:63-70. https://doi.org/10.1016/j.sleep.2016.06.018 (permission pending).)

An exciting and developing area of research in the management of refractory OSA in pediatric patients with DS is surgical implantation of a hypoglossal nerve stimulator. The device is surgically implanted in the chest, similar to a pacemaker device, and is powered on and off via remote control. It works by sensing upper airway obstruction and stimulating the hypoglossal nerve to contract the muscles of the tongue, thereby relieving the obstruction. While the clinical trials are still in progress, an update published in 2020 revealed promising early results. Twenty patients with DS (ages 10–21) with severe OSA despite AT, and inability to tolerate PAP, were evaluated. The study revealed an 85% reduction in AHI, 70% correction to at least mild OSA, and a median compliance of over 9 hours/night. There were no serious complications associated with the intervention. Four patients now have data for greater than 44 months and all participants have maintained a reduction of AHI by at least 50%.[45,46]

HEARING AND SPEECH
Anatomic Considerations

The ears of the DS patient have multiple typical morphologic characteristics. Previous studies have found that at birth, the pinna can be up to two standard deviations in size

A

Name of rater _____

Scoring template for pediatric sleep endoscopy

Indicate the greatest (box) and least (circle) obstructed views for each of the following locations:

Adenoid	0	1	2	3
Velum	0	1	2	3
LPW/tonsils	0	1	2	3
Tongue base	0	1	2	3
Supraglottis	0	1	2	3
Lingual tonsils	Present	Absent		

Adjunct airway needed for airway support?

Jaw thrust	Yes	No
Oral airway	Yes	No
Other (specify)		

Primary anesthetic used:	Propofol	Dexmedetomidine	Other
Reliability of examination:	Poor	Fair	Good

B

For each location, assess view obtained at the most and least obstructed points in respiratory cycle.

Adenoid: posterior view from nasal cavity

0 = Absent adenoids
1 = 0-50% Obstruction of choana
2 = 50%-99% Obstruction of choana
3 = Complete obstruction of choana

Velum: inferior view from nasopharynx; assessing anterior-posterior obstruction

0 = No obstruction (complete view of tongue base and/or larynx)
1 = 0-50% Anterior-posterior closure (some view of tongue base/larynx)
2 = 50%-99% Anterior-posterior closure (no view of tongue base/larynx, but not against posterior pharyngeal wall)
3 = Complete closure against posterior pharyngeal wall

Lateral pharyngeal wall: inferior view from velum; assessing lateral pharyngeal wall/tonsillar obstruction

0 = No obstruction
1 = 0-50% Lateral obstruction
2 = 50%-99% Lateral obstruction
3 = Complete obstruction

Tongue base: inferior view from oropharynx; assessing anterior-posterior obstruction

0 = No obstruction (complete view of vallecula)
1 = 0-50% Obstruction (vallecula not visible)
2 = 50%-99% Obstruction (epiglottis not contacting posterior pharyngeal wall)
3 = Complete obstruction (epiglottis against posterior pharyngeal wall)

Supraglottis: inferior view with tongue base (if obstructing) out of the way, with or without jaw thrust

0 = No obstruction (full view of vocal cords)
1 = 0-50% Obstruction (vocal cords partially obscured but >50% visible)
2 = 50%-99% Obstruction (>50% of vocal cords obscured)
3 = Complete obstruction (glottic opening not seen)

Fig. 4. Scoring template and representative photos for drug-induced sleep endoscopy. (*A*) Scoring template for pediatric drug-induced sleep endoscopy. (*B*) Site of obstruction and obstruction score with representative photos. LPW, Lateral Pharyngeal Wall. (*Data from* Chan DK, Liming BJ, Horn DL, Parikh SR. A new scoring system for upper airway pediatric sleep endoscopy. *JAMA Otolaryngol Head Neck Surg.* 2014;140(7):595-602. https://doi.org/10.1001/jamaoto.2014.612 (permission pending).)

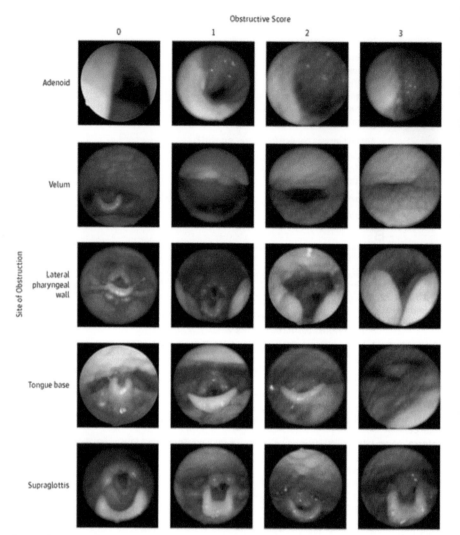

Fig. 4. (*continued*)

below that of the average newborn.[47] In addition, approximately 40% of patients with DS will also have stenotic external ear canals,[48] making ear examinations and the diagnosis of middle ear pathology difficult. The Eustachian tubes of patients with DS are also significantly narrower and more collapsed than in their nonsyndromic counterparts.[49] Together these factors greatly increase the incidence of Eustachian tube dysfunction in these patients.

Hearing loss in patients with DS can be conductive, sensorineural, or mixed in nature. Approximately 70% of patients with DS pass their newborn hearing screen.[50] However, almost 50% of patients with DS will be diagnosed with hearing loss, the majority of which is conductive in nature, secondary to middle ear effusions.[50] The rate of sensorineural hearing loss is significantly lower, only found in approximately 4% of these patients[50,51] and can be due to inner ear dysplasia.[52] An even smaller proportion of patients with DS will have a hearing loss that is mixed in nature.

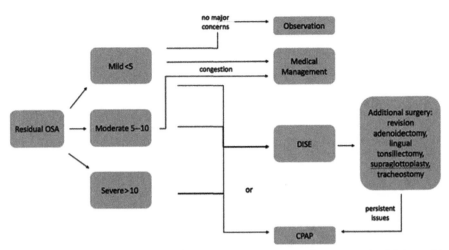

Fig. 5. Algorithm for the management of residual obstructive sleep apnea in children with Down syndrome after primary adenotonsillectomy. OSA, obstructive sleep apnea; DISE, drug-induced sleep endoscopy; CPAP, continuous positive airway pressure. (*Data from* Best J, Mutchnick S, Ida J, Billings KR. Trends in the management of obstructive sleep apnea in pediatric patients with Down syndrome. Int J Pediatr Otorhinolaryngol. 2018;110:1-5. https://doi.org/10.1016/j.ijporl.2018.04.008 (permission pending).)

Evaluation

Evaluation of the ears and hearing can take many forms. On the most basic level, a good otoscopic examination can provide vital information. However, given the propensity for ear canal stenosis in the patient with DS, this can prove to be difficult. If this cannot be performed, the American Academy of Pediatrics has recommended referral to an otolaryngologist for ear examinations every 3 to 6 months until the pediatrician is able to visualize the tympanic membrane and obtain reliable tympanometry.[53]

Beyond direct visualization of the ear, hearing evaluations also provide valuable information, and **Table 2** lists various options by age. All children should undergo newborn hearing screening by 1 month of age (Joint Committee on Infant Hearing). This initial evaluation can be either in the form of an auditory brainstem response (ABR) or otoacoustic emissions (OAE). Any child that refers on the newborn hearing screen needs to have confirmatory testing by 3 months, with the goal to begin appropriate intervention no later than 6 months of age.[53]

Recent studies have suggested that patients with DS may benefit from more frequent hearing evaluations even if they pass the newborn hearing screen. Given the high likelihood of developing middle ear effusions and conductive hearing loss, it has been suggested that it would be optimal to perform a natural sleep ABR by 3 months of age, even if the newborn hearing screen was normal.[54] If this evaluation is abnormal, further testing under sedation can be performed. This more frequent screening would help identify hearing loss at a younger age and guide hearing rehabilitation.

As the DS child ages, behavioral audiometry can often be performed to assess the hearing without sedation. Behavioral audiometry includes visual reinforcement audiometry, conditioned play audiometry, and conventional audiometry. With the typical child, reliable data can be obtained using behavioral audiometry starting at 6 months of age. For children with DS, this can be delayed significantly. Most children with DS

A Optimal Sedation for Pediatric DISE: Statements That Reached Consensus.

No.	Statements that reached consensus	Mean	Outliers
26	Either propofol or dexmedetomidine is an optimal form of sedation for use in pediatric DISE.	7.75	0
27	The level of sedation during pediatric DISE should be titrated to audible snoring, an obstructive breathing pattern, or both while allowing for flexible endoscopy without patient reactivity or awakening.	8.25	0
30	Inhalational agents may be used for induction and to gain intravenous access during DISE but should be discontinued for the diagnostic portion of the study.	8.50	0
31	The surgeon and anesthetist should agree on the sedation protocol prior to DISE.	9.00	0

B Grading/Interpretation of Pediatric DISE: Statements That Reached Consensus.

No.	Statements that reached consensus	Mean	Outliers
39	During pediatric DISE, the following parameters should be observed and documented for each anatomic level: (a) site, (b) pattern or shape, and (c) severity of obstruction.	8.75	0
40	During pediatric DISE, the following anatomic sites should be assessed and documented: nasal airway (including nasal cavities, nasopharynx), palate/velum, pharyngeal airway (including lateral oropharyngeal wall and tongue base), and supraglottic larynx.	8.86	0
48b	Cine MRI can be a useful adjuvant to DISE in children to determine the thickness of lingual tonsils and assess the contribution of the tongue base to palatal obstruction observed during DISE.	7.50	1

Fig. 6. (*A*) Various options are appropriate for pediatric drug-induced sleep endoscopy as long as a surgeon and anesthetist agree on protocol preoperatively. (*B*) It is critical that grading and interpretation of pediatric drug-induced sleep endoscopy assess various predetermined sites with anatomic descriptions documented. (*Data from* Baldassari, C.M., Lam, D.J., Ishman, S.L., Chernobilsky, B., Friedman, N.R., Giordano, T., Lawlor, C., Mitchell, R.B., Nardone, H., Ruda, J., Zalzal, H., Deneal, A., Dhepyasuwan, N., Rosenfeld, R.M., 2021. Expert Consensus Statement: Pediatric Drug-Induced Sleep Endoscopy. Otolaryngology–Head and Neck Surgery 165, 578–591. https://doi.org/10.1177/0194599820985000 (permission pending).)

will be able to obtain reliable behavioral testing at 16 months, but some can be delayed up to 30 months.[55] As a result, these children may require more frequent sedated examinations to monitor hearing.

Therapeutic Options

Once the type of hearing loss or ear issue has been established, the next step is to determine the appropriate therapeutic option.

For children with Eustachian tube dysfunction, chronic middle ear fluid, and associated conductive hearing loss, this frequently involves the placement of tympanostomy tubes to equalize the pressure of the middle ear and allow for drainage of the middle ear fluid. Studies of tympanostomy tube prevalence have found that children with DS have a 13-fold higher risk of needing pressure equalizing tubes between the ages of 3 to 5 when compared with their nonsyndromic counterparts.[56] Despite the higher likelihood of needing tympanostomy tubes, children with DS tend to have greater delays in having the tubes placed, likely due to delays in the diagnosis and management of comorbid conditions.[57] Additionally, these children are more likely to need multiple sets of ear tubes due to prolonged Eustachian tube dysfunction. Over 60% of patients with DS will need two or more sets of ear tubes.[58] Long term complications of ear tubes, including perforation, atelectasis, and acquired cholesteatoma, are common in these patients, particularly if they require 3 or more sets of ear tubes.[58]

If further hearing loss is detected beyond the Eustachian tube dysfunction, patients may need other technologies for hearing restoration. This can include conventional hearing aids as well as surgical implants. Conventional hearing aids are frequently difficult to use in young children and may be more difficult to tolerate in the DS child with learning difficulties.[6] Alternatives to conventional hearing aids can include the bone anchored hearing aid (BAHA) Softband or BAHA soundarc . These are nonsurgical solutions to improve bone conduction without having something directly in the ear, which many children find bothersome.

Should nonsurgical options be insufficient, there are multiple surgical options for hearing rehabilitation depending on the underlying cause and type of hearing loss. For patients with known middle ear pathology, which may be acquired from the underlying Eustachian tube dysfunction, surgical management with mastoidectomy and ossiculoplasty may be necessary. This can be difficult due to the persistent Eustachian tube dysfunction and frequently requires repeat procedures due to recurrent disease.[59] Even after this pathology is resolved, patients may still require adjunctive technologies to optimize the hearing.

Surgically placed bone-anchored hearing implants are indicated for conductive hearing loss, mixed hearing loss, and single-sided deafness. These come in multiple forms including percutaneous and magnetic versions. These depend on osseointegration into the skull to function properly. Previous studies have found these to be a good option for patients with DS with no increased complication rates and high patient and caregiver satisfaction rates.[60]

For patients with severe to profound sensorineural hearing loss or single-sided deafness, cochlear implantation is an option for hearing rehabilitation. Given the high rate of middle and inner ear malformations in these patients, detailed diagnostic imaging must be performed in the assessment of cochlear implant candidacy.[61] For those that are good candidates, the limited case studies have shown this to be a safe surgery with no increased risk of complication in this population.[62] It should be noted that language acquisition skills may still present differently in these patients despite cochlear implantation. Therefore, parents should be counseled appropriately and consider the development of alternative methods of communication with these patients.[61,63]

SPECIAL CONSIDERATIONS
Cervical Instability

It is estimated that more than 50% of children with DS have some variant of cervical instability due to a combination of increased ligamentous laxity and bony deformities.[64] Up to 30% of children with DS have atlanto-axial instability and anywhere from 10% to 60% have atlanto-occipital instability (depending on whether a 7 mm or a 4 mm occiputm-C1 subluxation radiological cutoff is used, respectively).[65] However, exact incidence is hard to establish, as the vast majority (98%–99%) of these patients are asymptomatic from this condition.[66] Symptoms to look out for can vary by age but would largely be symptoms expected with myelopathy such as neck pain/stiffness, abnormal head position, numbness/tingling, gait abnormalities, decreased upper extremity motor skills, changes in muscular tone, decreased coordination, or changes in bowel/bladder function.[64,67,68]

The AAP does not recommend routine screening imaging for asymptomatic patients, and there is currently no consensus regarding preoperative radiographic screening. Ultimately, the decision regarding whether to obtain preoperative imaging should be made on a case-by-case basis by the performing surgeon and anesthesiologist. The patient should undergo a thorough history and physical examination to screen the patient before undergoing any surgery, preferably by a physician who knows the patient well. If cervical instability screening is desired, a dynamic cervical spine radiograph is commonly used and allows for the evaluation under active, rather than passive, flexion. A lateral cervical spine radiograph is another commonly used option. MRIs and CTs can be used; however, they typically necessitate sedation and/or a higher radiation dose, and can only evaluate passive flexion. Of note, vertebral radiographs should not be used in patients under 3 year old, as there is not yet enough bone mineralization for adequate evaluation at that age and they have a low positive predictive value for developing cervical instability.[66,68,69]

Incidence of peri-operative cervical spinal cord injury is very low in patients with DS, with only a few cases described in the literature.[70] This is likely attributable to the fact that spinal cord injury from cervical instability is typically caused by flexion, rather than the extension positioning required for laryngoscopy. During laryngoscopy, special attention to cervical protection should be made with either manual in-line stabilization (MILS) or neck collars, with neck collars providing a good balance of cervical immobilization and less restriction of cervical extension.[65]

In patients with DS, it is advised to limit intraoperative head motion as much as possible, with repositioning the operating table, rather than the patient, and use of supports and straps as appropriate. It is also advised to perform most pediatric otolaryngology procedures, such as AT, in a neutral neck position, and if rotation is necessary (eg, myringotomy) that angle of rotation be $</=60°$.[64,65]

Intraoperative somatosensory evoked potentials (SEPs) are a newer technology that can detect delays in neural transmission suggestive of spinal cord compression. While it is not routinely used currently, SEP intraoperative monitoring may become more commonly used in patients with DS.[64]

Anesthesia

Patients with DS are likely to require at least one surgery under general anesthesia at some point in their lives and there are several risks associated with anesthesia that should be taken into consideration with surgical planning. Children with DS have higher rates of cardiac and pulmonary abnormalities such as CHD (commonly due to atrio-ventricular septal defect), lower airway abnormalities, and pulmonary hypertension.[7] Therefore, it is important to have anesthesiologists with a good understanding of the physiologic anomalies commonly seen in this patient population involved in their cases. In a study by Borland and colleagues, the most common anesthetic-related complications included bradycardia (which was severe in 3.66%), airway obstruction, difficult intubation, and postintubation croup.[71] Increased risks can occur even in the setting of short procedures. Due to these and other risks discussed later in discussion, it would be prudent to be judicious with surgical planning in these patients and combine procedures whereby appropriate to decrease the number of necessary endotracheal intubation events.

Children with DS have higher rates of postoperative obstructive breathing than children in the general population, with some postextubation stridor incidence estimates between 33% and 38%.[71–73] The reason for this is likely multifactorial. Children with DS are also known to have higher rates of OSA, stemming from anatomic variants including small midface, narrow nasopharynx, micrognathia, small larynx, and higher rates of obesity, as well as hypotonia and sleep-induced ventilatory dysfunction.[73,74]

While there is a move to perform more otolaryngologic procedures in the outpatient setting, this may not always be the most appropriate health care setting for pediatric patients with DS. For procedures requiring general endotracheal anesthesia, there are higher rates of postoperative respiratory complications in these children, and they have also been found to have delayed return to adequate oral intake.[71,72,74] For these reasons, it has been recommended that patients with DS undergoing procedures requiring intubation, particularly AT, should be admitted to the hospital for postoperative observation.

Along with other well-known anatomic differences in the head and neck observed in children with DS, it has also been shown that patients within this population have higher rates of congenital airway narrowing, involving both the subglottis and the trachea. This places children with DS at increased risk of developing subglottic stenosis from airway mucosal injury during endotracheal intubation.[73,75] Therefore, it is recommended to use endotracheal tubes at least 2 sizes smaller than what would be selected in a child without DS of the same age. Following endotracheal tube placement, it is important to confirm the appropriately sized tube has been selected for the patient. To evaluate this, an audible air leak should be present at an inspiratory pressure between 10 and 20 cm H_2O.[23]

Considerations with Bilateral Myringotomy and Tube Placement

Tympanostomy tube placement is the most commonly performed otolaryngologic procedure in patients with DS. One study estimated that these children had a 13.7 times higher risk of getting tympanostomy tube placement when compared with pediatric control.[56] When performing myringotomies with tympanostomy tube placement in children with DS, consideration should be made to use smaller tympanostomy tubes than one would typically choose for children of similar age and size.[6,7,56]

Bilateral myringotomy and tube (BMT) placement can be technically more difficult in this patient population due to stenotic external auditory canals, which pose a challenge to both visualization and instrument manipulation. A smaller tympanostomy tube may be more easily maneuvered through this tight anatomic space.[6]

These patients are also much more prone to dislodgement of tympanostomy tubes and complications from tympanostomy tube placement, most notably, TM perforations and cholesteatomas.[59] This is especially true in children who have had 3 sets or more of tympanostomy tubes. This is caused by an absent lamina propria layer, which normally would provide blood supply and supportive collagen fibers. The thinness and flaccidity of the tympanic membrane can often be appreciated on pneumatic otoscopy.[6,7]

Bone Anchored Hearing Aid Softband

As previously discussed, BAHA can be an effective option in children with DS and hearing loss who failed or are not candidates for more traditional treatments, such as in-ear hearing aids and BMT.[6,7] However, the manufacturer of the BAHA device only recommends its use in children over the age of 5.[60] There are higher rates of implant nonintegration in younger children, especially in those with bone thickness less than 2.5 mm.[60,76] An alternative to the implanted BAHA device in these children is a BAHA Softband, which integrates all of the components of the BAHA system into a single device housed in a soft headband. The BAHA Softband has been shown to have similar efficacy to the conventional BAHA device and aids in the pivotal speech and language development that occurs in children at these young ages.[77] The headband can also be fitted with 2 BAHA devices, so that bilateral hearing loss can successfully be addressed with this option.

Endocrinology

There is a well-established association between DS and thyroid dysfunction, with 28% to 40% of children with DS identified as having thyroid abnormalities. These estimates go up as the children age.[78,79] The thyroid abnormalities seen are primarily hypothyroidism caused by compensated hypothyroidism, congenital hypothyroidism, and Hashimoto's thyroiditis, of which compensated hypothyroidism (isolated elevated thyroid-stimulating hormone (TSH) in the setting of normal free thyroxine (fT4)) is the most common manifestation. Hyperthyroidism caused by Grave's disease has also been seen in this patient population, but is less commonly seen than hypothyroid states.[78,79]

It is recommended that neonates with DS get screened with TSH and fT4 levels shortly after birth, and the AAP amended their position in 2001 to recommend screening at ages 6 and 12 months, and annually thereafter.[79,80]

Untreated hypothyroidism may contribute to the body habitus differences that are observed in patients with DS, such as shorter stature and higher weight-to-length ratios and body mass indicies.[81] Short-term thyroxine supplementation has not been shown to have a significant effect on these children's growth or BMI. However, the effects of long-term supplementation have yet to be established.[79] Currently, thyroxine supplementation is not widely used.

Poor wound healing after surgery, such as higher rates of wound infection and wound dehiscence, in these children, has been documented, primarily in the orthopedic surgery literature.[82,83] Exact mechanisms to explain this phenomenon have not been elucidated in the literature.

Children with DS have higher rates of diabetes mellitus (1%) compared with the general pediatric population (0.25%).[78] Diabetes mellitus has been tied to poorer wound healing outcomes due to circulation impairments on the microvascular level. While this is certainly not a sufficient explanation for the poorer wound outcomes observed, it is a consideration to be made when proceeding with surgery in patients with DS and diabetes mellitus.

Inspire Clinical Trials

There is a There are clinical trials presently underway to assess the safety and efficacy of the Inspire hypoglossal nerve stimulator in use in pediatric patients with DS suffering from OSA. The device is surgically implanted in the chest, similar to a pacemaker device, and is powered on and off via remote control. It works by sensing upper airway obstruction and stimulating the hypoglossal nerve to contract the muscles of the tongue, thereby relieving the obstruction. While the clinical trials are still in progress, an update published in 2020 revealed early results showing promise. Looking at 20 children with DS and OSA who had failed therapy with AT and CPAP, there was an 85% reduction in AHI and a median compliance of over 9 hours/night. There were also no serious complications associated with the surgery or the therapy, and only 2 cases of minor adverse events that were successfully corrected with revision surgery.[45]

DISCLOSURE

The authors have nothing to disclose.

REFERENCES

1. Parker SE, Mai CT, Canfield MA, et al. Updated National Birth Prevalence estimates for selected birth defects in the United States, 2004-2006. Birth Defects Res A Clin Mol Teratol 2010;88(12):1008–16.
2. Bull MJ, Committee on Genetics. Health supervision for children with Down syndrome [published correction appears in Pediatrics 2011;128(2):393–406.
3. Patel TA, Nguyen SA, White DR. Down Syndrome as an indicator for pediatric otolaryngologic procedures. Int J Pediatr Otorhinolaryngol 2018;112:182–7.
4. Bassett EC, Musso MF. Otolaryngologic management of Down syndrome patients: what is new? Curr Opin Otolaryngol Head Neck Surg 2017;25(6):493–7.

5. Chin CJ, Khami MM, Husein M. A general review of the otolaryngologic manifestations of Down Syndrome. Int J Pediatr Otorhinolaryngol 2014;78(6):899–904.

6. Ramia M, Musharrafieh U, Khaddage W, et al. Revisiting Down syndrome from the ENT perspective: review of literature and recommendations. Eur Arch Otorhinolaryngol 2014;271(5):863–9.

7. Rodman R, Pine HS. The otolaryngologist's approach to the patient with Down syndrome. Otolaryngol Clin North Am 2012;45(3):599–viii.

8. Weijerman ME, van Furth AM, van der Mooren MD, et al. Prevalence of congenital heart defects and persistent pulmonary hypertension of the neonate with Down syndrome. Eur J Pediatr 2010;169(10):1195–9.

9. Vicente A, Bravo-González LA, López-Romero A, et al. Craniofacial morphology in down syndrome: a systematic review and meta-analysis. Sci Rep 2020;10(1): 19895. Published 2020 Nov 16.

10. Allareddy V, Ching N, Macklin EA, et al. Craniofacial features as assessed by lateral cephalometric measurements in children with Down syndrome. Prog Orthod 2016;17(1):35.

11. Starbuck JM, Cole TM 3rd, Reeves RH, et al. The Influence of trisomy 21 on facial form and variability. Am J Med Genet A 2017;173(11):2861–72.

12. Maris M, Verhulst S, Wojciechowski M, et al. Prevalence of Obstructive Sleep Apnea in Children with Down Syndrome. Sleep 2016;39(3):699–704. Published 2016 Mar 1.

13. Narawane A, Eng J, Rappazzo C, et al. Airway protection & patterns of dysphagia in infants with down syndrome: Videofluoroscopic swallow study findings & correlations. Int J Pediatr Otorhinolaryngol 2020;132:109908.

14. Knollman PD, Heubi CH, Wiley S, et al. Demographic and Clinical Characteristics Associated With Adherence to Guideline-Based Polysomnography in Children With Down Syndrome. Otolaryngol Head Neck Surg 2021;164(4):877–83.

15. Esbensen AJ, Beebe DW, Byars KC, et al. Use of Sleep Evaluations and Treatments in Children with Down Syndrome. J Dev Behav Pediatr 2016;37(8):629–36.

16. Hamilton J, Yaneza MM, Clement WA, et al. The prevalence of airway problems in children with Down's syndrome. Int J Pediatr Otorhinolaryngol 2016;81:1–4.

17. Vielkind M, Wolter-Warmerdam K, Jackson A, et al. Airway obstruction and inflammation on combined bronchoscopy in children with Down syndrome. Pediatr Pulmonol 2021;56(9):2932–9.

18. Cockerill CC, Frisch CD, Rein SE, et al. Supraglottoplasty outcomes in children with Down syndrome. Int J Pediatr Otorhinolaryngol 2016;87:87–90.

19. Salloum S, Mahsoun Y, Al-Khatib T, et al. Supraglottoplasty in the management of laryngomalacia in children with down syndrome: A systematic review. Int J Pediatr Otorhinolaryngol 2021;142:110630.

20. De Lausnay M, Verhulst S, Boel L, et al. The prevalence of lower airway anomalies in children with Down syndrome compared to controls. Pediatr Pulmonol 2020; 55(5):1259–63.

21. De Lausnay M, Ides K, Wojciechowski M, et al. Pulmonary complications in children with Down syndrome: A scoping review [published online ahead of print, 2021 May 5]. Paediatr Respir Rev 2021. https://doi.org/10.1016/j.prrv.2021.04. 006. S1526-0542(21)00029-34.

22. Fockens MM, Hölscher M, Limpens J, et al. Tracheal anomalies associated with Down syndrome: A systematic review. Pediatr Pulmonol 2021;56(5):814–22.

23. Shott SR. Down syndrome: analysis of airway size and a guide for appropriate intubation. Laryngoscope 2000;110(4):585–92.

24. Okamoto T, Nishijima E, Maruo A, et al. Congenital tracheal stenosis: the prognostic significance of associated cardiovascular anomalies and the optimal timing of surgical treatment. J Pediatr Surg 2009;44(2):325–8.
25. Skotko BG, Macklin EA, Muselli M, et al. A predictive model for obstructive sleep apnea and Down syndrome. Am J Med Genet A 2017;173(4):889–96.
26. Maris M, Verhulst S, Saldien V, et al. Drug-induced sedation endoscopy in surgically naive children with Down syndrome and obstructive sleep apnea. Sleep Med 2016;24:63–70.
27. Akkina SR, Ma CC, Kirkham EM, et al. Does drug induced sleep endoscopy-directed surgery improve polysomnography measures in children with Down Syndrome and obstructive sleep apnea? Acta Otolaryngol 2018;138(11):1009–13.
28. Hyzer JM, Milczuk HA, Macarthur CJ, et al. Drug-Induced Sleep Endoscopy Findings in Children With Obstructive Sleep Apnea With vs Without Obesity or Down Syndrome. JAMA Otolaryngol Head Neck Surg 2021;147(2):175–81.
29. Jackson A, Maybee J, Wolter-Warmerdam K, et al. Associations between age, respiratory comorbidities, and dysphagia in infants with down syndrome. Pediatr Pulmonol 2019;54(11):1853–9.
30. Stanley MA, Shepherd N, Duvall N, et al. Clinical identification of feeding and swallowing disorders in 0-6 month old infants with Down syndrome. Am J Med Genet A 2019;179(2):177–82.
31. Farpour HR, Moosavi SA, Mohammadian Z, et al. Comparing the tongue and lip strength and Endurance of children with down syndrome with their typical Peers using IOPI. Dysphagia 2021. https://doi.org/10.1007/s00455-021-10359-4.
32. Hamill CS, Tracy MM, Staggs VS, et al. Tracheostomy in the pediatric trisomy 21 population. Int J Pediatr Otorhinolaryngol 2021;140:110540.
33. Nation J, Brigger M. The Efficacy of Adenotonsillectomy for Obstructive Sleep Apnea in Children with Down Syndrome: A Systematic Review. Otolaryngol Head Neck Surg 2017;157(3):401–8.
34. Thottam PJ, Trivedi S, Siegel B, et al. Comparative outcomes of severe obstructive sleep apnea in pediatric patients with Trisomy 21. Int J Pediatr Otorhinolaryngol 2015;79(7):1013–6.
35. Best J, Mutchnick S, Ida J, et al. Trends in management of obstructive sleep apnea in pediatric patients with Down syndrome. Int J Pediatr Otorhinolaryngol 2018;110:1–5.
36. Raposo D, Menezes M, Rito J, et al. Predictors of OSA following adenotonsillectomy in children with trisomy 21. Clin Otolaryngol 2021;46(1):256–62.
37. Cottrell J, Zahr SK, Propst EJ, et al. Morbidity and mortality from adenotonsillectomy in children with trisomy 21. Int J Pediatr Otorhinolaryngol 2020;138:110377.
38. Wootten CT, Chinnadurai S, Goudy SL. Beyond adenotonsillectomy: outcomes of sleep endoscopy-directed treatments in pediatric obstructive sleep apnea. Int J Pediatr Otorhinolaryngol 2014;78(7):1158–62.
39. Mahmoud M, Ishman SL, McConnell K, et al. Upper Airway Reflexes are Preserved During Dexmedetomidine Sedation in Children With Down Syndrome and Obstructive Sleep Apnea. J Clin Sleep Med 2017;13(5):721–7.
40. Propst EJ, Amin R, Talwar N, et al. Midline posterior glossectomy and lingual tonsillectomy in obese and nonobese children with down syndrome: Biomarkers for success. Laryngoscope 2017;127(3):757–63.
41. Prosser JD, Shott SR, Rodriguez O, et al. Polysomnographic outcomes following lingual tonsillectomy for persistent obstructive sleep apnea in down syndrome. Laryngoscope 2017;127(2):520–4.

42. Verhulst S. Long Term Continuous Positive Airway Pressure and Non-invasive Ventilation in Obstructive Sleep Apnea in Children With Obesity and Down Syndrome. Front Pediatr 2020;8:534.
43. Hurvitz MS, Lesser DJ, Dever G, et al. Findings of routine nocturnal polysomnography in children with Down syndrome: a retrospective cohort study. Sleep Med 2020;76:58–64.
44. Gray AJ, Nielsen KR, Ellington LE, et al. Tracheal pressure generated by high-flow nasal cannula in 3D-Printed pediatric airway models. Int J Pediatr Otorhinolaryngol 2021;145:110719.
45. Caloway CL, Diercks GR, Keamy D, et al. Update on hypoglossal nerve stimulation in children with down syndrome and obstructive sleep apnea. Laryngoscope 2020;130(4):E263–7.
46. Stenerson ME, Yu PK, Kinane TB, et al. Long-term stability of hypoglossal nerve stimulation for the treatment of obstructive sleep apnea in children with Down syndrome. Int J Pediatr Otorhinolaryngol 2021;149:110868.
47. Schwartz DM, Schwartz RH. Acoustic impedance and otoscopic findings in young children with Down's syndrome. Arch Otolaryngol 1978;104(11):652–6.
48. Strome M. Down's syndrome: a modern otorhinolaryngological perspective. Laryngoscope 1981;91(10):1581–94.
49. Shibahara Y, Sando I. Congenital anomalies of the eustachian tube in Down syndrome. Histopathologic case report. Ann Otol Rhinol Laryngol 1989;98(7 Pt 1):543–7.
50. Park AH, Wilson MA, Stevens PT, et al. Identification of hearing loss in pediatric patients with Down syndrome. Otolaryngol Head Neck Surg 2012;146(1):135–40.
51. De Schrijver L, Topsakal V, Wojciechowski M, et al. Prevalence and etiology of sensorineural hearing loss in children with down syndrome: A cross-sectional study. Int J Pediatr Otorhinolaryngol 2019;116:168–72.
52. Blaser S, Propst EJ, Martin D, et al. Inner ear dysplasia is common in children with Down syndrome (trisomy 21). Laryngoscope 2006;116(12):2113–9.
53. American Academy of Pediatrics, Joint Committee on Infant Hearing. Year 2007 position statement: Principles and guidelines for early hearing detection and intervention programs. Pediatrics 2007;120(4):898–921.
54. Basonbul RA, Ronner EA, Rong A, et al. Audiologic testing in children with Down Syndrome: Are current guidelines optimal? Int J Pediatr Otorhinolaryngol 2020;134:110017.
55. Nightengale EE, Wolter-Warmerdam K, Yoon PJ, et al. Behavioral Audiology Procedures in Children With Down Syndrome. Am J Audiol 2020;29(3):356–64.
56. Bernardi GF, Pires CTF, Oliveira NP, et al. Prevalence of pressure equalization tube placement and hearing loss in children with down syndrome. Int J Pediatr Otorhinolaryngol 2017;98:48–52.
57. Bachrach K, Bains A, Shehan JN, et al. Barriers to timely tympanostomy tube placement in trisomy 21. Int J Pediatr Otorhinolaryngol 2021;140:110516.
58. Paulson LM, Weaver TS, Macarthur CJ. Outcomes of tympanostomy tube placement in children with Down syndrome–a retrospective review. Int J Pediatr Otorhinolaryngol 2014;78(2):223–6.
59. Ghadersohi S, Bhushan B, Billings KR. Challenges and outcomes of cholesteatoma management in children with Down syndrome. Int J Pediatr Otorhinolaryngol 2018;106:80–4.

60. McDermott AL, Williams J, Kuo MJ, et al. The role of bone anchored hearing aids in children with Down syndrome. Int J Pediatr Otorhinolaryngol 2008;72(6):751–7.

61. Clarós P, Remjasz A, Clarós-Pujol A, et al. Long-term Outcomes in Down Syndrome Children After Cochlear Implantation: Particular Issues and Considerations. Otol Neurotol 2019;40(10):1278–86.

62. Hans PS, England R, Prowse S, et al. UK and Ireland experience of cochlear implants in children with Down syndrome. Int J Pediatr Otorhinolaryngol 2010;74(3):260–4.

63. Heldahl MG, Eksveen B, Bunne M. Cochlear implants in eight children with Down Syndrome - Auditory performance and challenges in assessment. Int J Pediatr Otorhinolaryngol 2019;126:109636.

64. Bertolizio G, Saint-Martin C, Ingelmo P. Cervical instability in patients with Trisomy 21: The eternal gamble. Paediatr Anaesth 2018;28(10):830–3.

65. Hata T, Todd MM. Cervical spine considerations when anesthetizing patients with Down syndrome. Anesthesiology 2005;102(3):680–5.

66. Nakamura N, Inaba Y, Aota Y, et al. New radiological parameters for the assessment of atlantoaxial instability in children with Down syndrome: the normal values and the risk of spinal cord injury. Bone Joint J 2016;98-B(12):1704–10.

67. Pizzutillo PD, Herman MJ. Cervical spine issues in Down syndrome. J Pediatr Orthop 2005;25(2):253–9.

68. Hankinson TC, Anderson RC. Craniovertebral junction abnormalities in Down syndrome. Neurosurgery 2010;66(3 Suppl):32–8.

69. Lewanda AF, Matisoff A, Revenis M, et al. Preoperative evaluation and comprehensive risk assessment for children with Down syndrome. Paediatr Anaesth 2016;26(4):356–62.

70. Dedlow ER, Siddiqi S, Fillipps DJ, et al. Symptomatic atlantoaxial instability in an adolescent with trisomy 21 (Down's syndrome). Clin Pediatr (Phila) 2013;52(7):633–8.

71. Borland LM, Colligan J, Brandom BW. Frequency of anesthesia-related complications in children with Down syndrome under general anesthesia for noncardiac procedures. Paediatr Anaesth 2004;14(9):733–8.

72. Marcus CL, Keens TG, Bautista DB, et al. Obstructive sleep apnea in children with Down syndrome. Pediatrics 1991;88(1):132–9.

73. Kanamori G, Witter M, Brown J, et al. Otolaryngologic manifestations of Down syndrome. Otolaryngol Clin North Am 2000;33(6):1285–92.

74. Mitchell RB, Call E, Kelly J. Ear, nose and throat disorders in children with Down syndrome. Laryngoscope 2003;113(2):259–63.

75. Miller R, Gray SD, Cotton RT, et al. Subglottic stenosis and Down syndrome. Am J Otol 1990;11(4):274–7.

76. Tjellström A, Håkansson B, Granström G. Bone-anchored hearing aids: current status in adults and children. Otolaryngol Clin North Am 2001;34(2):337–64.

77. Hol MK, Cremers CW, Coppens-Schellekens W, et al. The BAHA Softband. A new treatment for young children with bilateral congenital aural atresia. Int J Pediatr Otorhinolaryngol 2005;69(7):973–80.

78. Roizen NJ, Patterson D. Down's syndrome. Lancet 2003;361(9365):1281–9.

79. Erlichman I, Mimouni FB, Erlichman M, et al. Thyroxine-Based Screening for Congenital Hypothyroidism in Neonates with Down Syndrome. J Pediatr 2016;173:165–8.

80. American Academy of Pediatrics. Committee on Genetics. American Academy of Pediatrics: Health supervision for children with Down syndrome. Pediatrics 2001;107(2):442–9.

81. Zemel BS, Pipan M, Stallings VA, et al. Growth Charts for Children With Down Syndrome in the United States. Pediatrics 2015;136(5):e1204–11.
82. Caird MS, Wills BP, Dormans JP. Down syndrome in children: the role of the orthopaedic surgeon. J Am Acad Orthop Surg 2006;14(11):610–9.
83. Mik G, Gholve PA, Scher DM, et al. Down syndrome: orthopedic issues. Curr Opin Pediatr 2008;20(1):30–6.

Moving?

Make sure your subscription moves with you!

To notify us of your new address, find your **Clinics Account Number** (located on your mailing label above your name), and contact customer service at:

Email: journalscustomerservice-usa@elsevier.com

800-654-2452 (subscribers in the U.S. & Canada)
314-447-8871 (subscribers outside of the U.S. & Canada)

Fax number: 314-447-8029

Elsevier Health Sciences Division
Subscription Customer Service
3251 Riverport Lane
Maryland Heights, MO 63043

*To ensure uninterrupted delivery of your subscription, please notify us at least 4 weeks in advance of move.

9780323848725